NATIONAL ACADEMIES
Sciences
Engineering
Medicine

NATIONAL
ACADEMIES
PRESS
Washington, DC

Realizing the Potential of Genomics across the Continuum of Precision Health Care

Theresa M. Wizemann,
Kathryn Asalone,
Meredith Hackmann, and
Sarah Beachy, *Rapporteurs*

Roundtable on Genomics
and Precision Health

Board on Health Sciences Policy

National Cancer Policy Forum

Board on Health Care Services

Health and Medicine Division

T0002901

Proceedings of a Workshop

NATIONAL ACADEMIES PRESS 500 Fifth Street, NW Washington, DC 20001

This activity was supported by contracts between the National Academy of Sciences and Air Force Medical Service (Contract No. FA8052-17-P-0007); Centers for Disease Control and Prevention (Contract No. 75D30121D11240, Task Order No. 75D30121F00002); Health Resources and Services Administration (Contract No. HHSH250201500001I, Task Order No. 75R60220F34021); National Institutes of Health (Contract No. HHSN263201800029I, Task Order Nos. HHSN26300010 and HHSN26300008): All of Us Research Program, National Cancer Institute, National Human Genome Research Institute, National Institute of Mental Health, National Institute of Nursing Research, and National Institute on Aging; 23andMe, Inc.; American Academy of Nursing; American Association for Cancer Research; American Cancer Society; American College of Medical Genetics and Genomics; American College of Radiology; American Medical Association; American Society of Clinical Oncology; American Society of Human Genetics; Association for Molecular Pathology; Association of American Cancer Institutes; Association of Community Cancer Centers; Biogen; Blue Cross and Blue Shield Association; Bristol Myers Squibb; Cancer Support Community; College of American Pathologists; Eisai Inc.; Flatiron Health; Geisinger; Genome Medical, Inc.; Helix; Illumina, Inc.; The Jackson Laboratory (JAX); Kaiser Foundation Health Plan, Inc.; Merck & Co., Inc.; Myriad Genetics; National Comprehensive Cancer Network; National Patient Advocate Foundation; National Society of Genetic Counselors; Novartis Oncology; Oncology Nursing Society; Partners in Health; Pfizer, Inc.; Regeneron; Sanofi; Society for Immunotherapy of Cancer; The University of Vermont Health Network Medical Group; University of California, San Francisco; and Vibrent Health. Any opinions, findings, conclusions, or recommendations expressed in this publication do not necessarily reflect the views of any organization or agency that provided support for the project.

International Standard Book Number-13: 978-0-309-70115-0
International Standard Book Number-10: 0-309-70115-5
Digital Object Identifier: https://doi.org/10.17226/26917

This publication is available from the National Academies Press, 500 Fifth Street, NW, Keck 360, Washington, DC 20001; (800) 624-6242 or (202) 334-3313; http://www.nap.edu.

Suggested citation: National Academies of Sciences, Engineering, and Medicine. 2023. *Realizing the potential of genomics across the continuum of precision health care: Proceedings of a workshop.* Washington, DC: The National Academies Press. https://doi.org/10.17226/26917.

The **National Academy of Sciences** was established in 1863 by an Act of Congress, signed by President Lincoln, as a private, nongovernmental institution to advise the nation on issues related to science and technology. Members are elected by their peers for outstanding contributions to research. Dr. Marcia McNutt is president.

The **National Academy of Engineering** was established in 1964 under the charter of the National Academy of Sciences to bring the practices of engineering to advising the nation. Members are elected by their peers for extraordinary contributions to engineering. Dr. John L. Anderson is president.

The **National Academy of Medicine** (formerly the Institute of Medicine) was established in 1970 under the charter of the National Academy of Sciences to advise the nation on medical and health issues. Members are elected by their peers for distinguished contributions to medicine and health. Dr. Victor J. Dzau is president.

The three Academies work together as the **National Academies of Sciences, Engineering, and Medicine** to provide independent, objective analysis and advice to the nation and conduct other activities to solve complex problems and inform public policy decisions. The National Academies also encourage education and research, recognize outstanding contributions to knowledge, and increase public understanding in matters of science, engineering, and medicine.

Learn more about the National Academies of Sciences, Engineering, and Medicine at **www.nationalacademies.org**.

PLANNING COMMITTEE ON REALIZING THE POTENTIAL OF GENOMICS ACROSS THE CONTINUUM OF PRECISION HEALTH CARE[1]

MIRA IRONS (*Cochair*), President and CEO, College of Physicians of Philadelphia

CHRISTA LESE MARTIN (*Cochair*), Chief Scientific Officer and Director, Autism and Developmental Medicine Institute, Geisinger

GWEN DARIEN, Executive Vice President for Patient Advocacy and Engagement, National Patient Advocate Foundation

W. GREGORY FEERO, Professor, Department of Community and Family Medicine, Geisel School of Medicine, Maine Dartmouth Family Medicine Residency Program, *representing JAMA*

ALISHA KEEHN, Branch Chief, Genetic Services Branch, Division of Services for Children with Special Health Needs, Maternal and Child Health Bureau, Health Resources and Services Administration

GABRIEL LÁZARO-MUÑOZ, Assistant Professor of Psychiatry, Harvard Medical School

OLUFUNMILAYO I. OLOPADE, Walter L. Palmer Distinguished Service, Professor of Medicine, University of Chicago

VICTORIA M. PRATT, Vice President, Molecular Diagnostics Quality Assessments, Optum Genomics, *representing Association for Molecular Pathology*

LAWRENCE M. SIMON, Medical Director for Utilization Management and Coding and Reimbursement, Blue Cross and Blue Shield of Louisiana

SARAH WORDSWORTH, Professor and University Lecturer, Health Economics Research Centre, Nuffield Department of Population Health, University of Oxford

Roundtable on Genomics and Precision Health Staff

SARAH BEACHY, Senior Program Officer and Roundtable Director
KATHRYN ASALONE, Associate Program Officer
MEREDITH HACKMANN, Associate Program Officer
LYDIA TEFERRA, Research Associate
APARNA CHERAN, Senior Program Assistant *(from June 2022)*

---

[1]The National Academies of Sciences, Engineering, and Medicine's planning committees are solely responsible for organizing the workshop, identifying topics, and choosing speakers. The responsibility for the published Proceedings of a Workshop rests with the workshop rapporteurs and the institution.

ROUNDTABLE ON GENOMICS AND PRECISION HEALTH[1]

W. GREGORY FEERO, Professor, Department of Community and Family Medicine, Geisel School of Medicine, Maine Dartmouth Family Medicine Residency Program, *representing JAMA*

MICHELLE PENNY, Executive Vice President, Research and Development, Embark Inc.

NAOMI ARONSON, Executive Director, Clinical Effectiveness and Policy, BlueCross BlueShield Association

ARIS BARAS, Senior Vice President, Regeneron Pharmaceuticals, General Manager, Regeneron Genetics Center

VENCE BONHAM JR., Acting Deputy Director, National Human Genome Research Institute

BERNICE COLEMAN, Director, Nursing Research Department, Performance Improvement Department, Nurse Practitioner, Heart Transplantation and Mechanical Circulatory Support Programs

ROBERT B. DARNELL, Heilbrunn Professor and Senior Physician Head, Laboratory of Molecular Neuro-Oncology, The Rockefeller University, Investigator, Howard Hughes Medical Institute, Founding Director and CEO Emeritus, New York Genome Center

GEOFFREY GINSBURG, Chief Medical and Science Officer, All of Us Research Program, National Institutes of Health, *representing Global Genomic Medicine Consortium*

JENNIFER GOLDSACK, Executive Director, Digital Medicine Society

JILL HAGENKORD, Chief Medical Officer, Optum Genomics

CASSIE HAJEK, Medical Director, Helix

RICHARD J. HODES, Director, National Institute on Aging, National Institutes of Health

GEOFF HOLLETT, Senior Science Policy Analyst, American Medical Association

MIRA IRONS, President and CEO, College of Physicians of Philadelphia

PRADUMAN JAIN, Chief Executive Officer, Vibrent Health

SEKAR KATHIRESAN, Director, Center for Genomic Medicine, Massachusetts General Hospital; Chief Executive Officer and Founder, Verve Therapeutics

ALISHA KEEHN, Branch Chief, Genetic Services Branch, Division of Services for Children with Special Health Needs, Maternal and Child Health Bureau, Health Resources and Services Administration (*from January 2022*)

---

[1] The National Academies of Sciences, Engineering, and Medicine's forums and roundtables do not issue, review, or approve individual documents. The responsibility for the published Proceedings of a Workshop rests with the workshop rapporteurs and the institution.

MUIN KHOURY, Director, Office of Public Health Genomics, Centers for Disease Control and Prevention

CHARLES LEE, Scientific Director and Professor, The Jackson Laboratory for Genomic Medicine

CHRISTA LESE MARTIN, Chief Scientific Officer, Director, Autism and Developmental Medicine Institute, Geisinger

MONA MILLER, Chief Executive Officer, American Society of Human Genetics

ADELE MITCHELL, Head of Clinical Genetics, Biogen

JENNIFER MOSER, Genomic Medicine Program, Office of Research and Development, U.S. Department of Veterans Affairs

MAXIMILIAN MUENKE, Chief Executive Officer, American College of Medical Genetics and Genomics

KENNETH OFFIT, Chief of Clinical Genetics Service, Robert and Kate Neihaus Chair in Inherited Cancer Genomics, and Vice Chair of Academic Affairs, Department of Medicine, Memorial Sloan Kettering Cancer Center; *representing American Society of Clinical Oncology*

KATHRYN PHILLIPS, Professor of Health and Economics and Health Services Research and Founding Director, Center for Translational and Policy Research on Precision Medicine, University of California, San Francisco

VICTORIA PRATT, Vice President, Molecular Diagnostics Quality Assessments, Optum Genomics, *representing Association for Molecular Pathology*

MURRAY ROSS, Vice President, Kaiser Foundation Health Plan, Inc.

WENDY RUBINSTEIN, Director, Personalized Medicine, Food and Drug Administration

NADEEM SARWAR, President, Eisai AiM Institute

SHERI SCHULLY, Deputy Chief Medical and Scientific Officer, All of Us Research Program, National Institutes of Health

JOAN SCOTT, Director, Division of Services for Children with Special Health Needs, Maternal and Child Health Bureau, Health Resources and Services Administration (*until January 2022*)

GEETHA SENTHIL, Program Officer, National Institute of Mental Health, National Institutes of Health

NONNIEKAYE SHELBURNE, Program Director, Clinical and Translational Epidemiology Branch, National Cancer Institute

NIKOLETTA SIDIROPOULOS, Medical Director of Genomic Medicine, Associate Professor of Pathology and Laboratory Medicine, University of Vermont Health Network, Larner College of Medicine at the University of Vermont

KATHERINE JOHANSEN TABER, Vice President, Clinical Product Research and Partnerships, Myriad Genetics

RYAN TAFT, Vice President, Scientific Research, Illumina

JACQUELYN TAYLOR, Professor of Nursing, Director, Center for Research on People of Color, Columbia University School of Nursing

SHARON TERRY, President and CEO, Genetic Alliance

JOYCE TUNG, Vice President, Research, 23andMe

JAMESON D. VOSS, Major, USAF, MC, FS, Chief, AFMS Precision Medicine, Air Force Medical Support Agency

KAREN WECK, Professor of Pathology and Laboratory Medicine, Professor of Clinical Genetics, University of North Carolina at Chapel Hill, *representing the College of American Pathologists*

CATHERINE A. WICKLUND, Director, Graduate Program in Genetic Counseling, Past President, National Society of Genetic Counselors, Associate Professor, Department of Obstetrics and Gynecology, Feinberg School of Medicine, Center for Genetic Medicine, Northwestern University

HUNTINGTON F. WILLARD, Chief Scientific Officer, Genome Medical, Inc.

SARAH WORDSWORTH, Professor and University Lecturer, Health Economics Research Centre, Nuffield Department of Population Health, University of Oxford

SHANNON ZENK, Director, National Institutes of Nursing Research

Reviewers

This Proceedings of a Workshop was reviewed in draft form by individuals chosen for their diverse perspectives and technical expertise. The purpose of this independent review is to provide candid and critical comments that will assist the National Academies of Sciences, Engineering, and Medicine in making each published proceedings as sound as possible and to ensure that it meets the institutional standards for quality, objectivity, evidence, and responsiveness to the charge. The review comments and draft manuscript remain confidential to protect the integrity of the process.

We thank the following individuals for their review of this proceedings:

JONATHAN BERG, M.D., PH.D., University of North Carolina at Chapel Hill
IAN CHUANG, M.D., M.S., Mercer

Although the reviewers listed above provided many constructive comments and suggestions, they were not asked to endorse the content of the proceedings nor did they see the final draft before its release. The review of this proceedings was overseen by **DANIEL R. MASYS, M.D.,** University of Washington. He was responsible for making certain that an independent examination of this proceedings was carried out in accordance with standards of the National Academies and that all review comments were carefully considered. Responsibility for the final content rests entirely with the rapporteurs and the National Academies. We also thank staff member Daniel Talmage for reading and providing helpful comments on this manuscript.

Acknowledgments

The support of the Roundtable on Genomics and Precision Health was crucial to the planning and conduct of this workshop, Realizing the Potential of Genomics across the Continuum of Precision Health Care. Federal sponsors for the workshop were the U.S. Air Force Medical Service, the Health Resources and Services Administration, and the following National Institutes of Health: the National Cancer Institute, the National Human Genome Research Institute, the National Institute on Aging, the National Institute of Mental Health, and the National Institute of Nursing Research, as well as the National Institutes of Health's All of Us Research Program. Nonfederal sponsorship was provided by 23andMe; American Academy of Nursing; American College of Medical Genetics and Genomics; American Medical Association; American Society of Clinical Oncology; Association for Molecular Pathology; Biogen; Blue Cross and Blue Shield Association; College of American Pathologists; Eisai, Inc.; Geisinger; Genome Medical, Inc.; Helix; Illumina, Inc.; The Jackson Laboratory; Kaiser Foundation Health Plan, Inc.; Myriad Genetics; National Society of Genetic Counselors; Regeneron Pharmaceuticals; University of Vermont Health Network Medical Group; University of California, San Francisco; and Vibrent Health.

Support from the many annual sponsors of the National Academies of Sciences, Engineering, and Medicine's National Cancer Policy Forum is crucial to the work of the forum. Federal sponsors include the Centers for Disease Control and Prevention and the National Cancer Institute/National Institutes of Health. Nonfederal sponsors include the American Association for Cancer Research, American Cancer Society, American College of Radiology,

American Society of Clinical Oncology, Association of American Cancer Institutes, Association of Community Cancer Centers, Bristol Myers Squibb, Cancer Support Community, Flatiron Health, Merck & Co., Inc., National Comprehensive Cancer Network, National Patient Advocate Foundation, Novartis Oncology, Oncology Nursing Society, Partners in Health, Pfizer Inc., Sanofi, and Society for Immunotherapy of Cancer.

The Roundtable on Genomics and Precision Health is grateful for the opportunity to collaborate with the National Cancer Policy Forum on this workshop. The Roundtable on Genomics and Precision Health wishes to express gratitude to the members of the planning committee for their work in developing an excellent workshop agenda and to the expert speakers who explored barriers and opportunities for improving adoption of genomics in clinical care. The project director would like to thank the project staff who worked diligently to develop both the workshop and the resulting proceedings.

Contents

Boxes and Figure

BOXES

FIGURE

Acronyms and Abbreviations

ACCE   analytic validity, clinical validity, clinical utility, and associated
            ethical, legal, and social implications
ACMG   American College of Medical Genetics and Genomics
ACT   ACTion
AI   artificial intelligence

CLIA   Clinical Laboratory Improvement Amendments
CMS   Centers for Medicare & Medicaid Services
CPIC   Clinical Pharmacogenetics Implementation Consortium
CPT®   Current Procedural Terminology
COVID-19   coronavirus disease of 2019

DNA   deoxyribonucleic acid

EHR   electronic health record

FBGRI   Faith-Based Genetic Research Institute
FDA   U.S. Food and Drug Administration

GINA   Genetic Information Nondiscrimination Act
GSP   genomic sequencing procedure
GWAS   genome-wide association studies

HLA   human leukocyte antigen

InheRET   Inherited Risk Evaluation Tool

LDT   laboratory-developed test
LGBTQ   lesbian, gay, bisexual, transgender, queer

MAC   Medicare Administrative Contractor
MCIT   Medicare Coverage for Innovative Technology
MEN   multiple endocrine neoplasia
mRNA   messenger RNA
MVP   Million Veteran Program

NGS   National Government Services
NHS   National Health Service (UK)
NICU   neonatal intensive care unit
NIH   National Institutes of Health

PCR   polymerase chain reaction
PLA   proprietary laboratory analysis
PTO   paid time off
PWS   Prader-Willi syndrome

RNA   ribonucleic acid

STEM   science, technology, engineering, and math

UCLA   University of California, Los Angeles
UK   United Kingdom
UPMC   University of Pittsburgh Medical Center

VA   Department of Veterans Affairs
VUS   variant of uncertain or unknown significance

1

Introduction[1]

Genomic testing is increasingly being applied in clinical practice to assess the risk or presence of disease and to guide prevention approaches and treatment decisions. The potential applications and benefits of genomic sequencing across the life span are many; however, obstacles to widespread adoption and integration of genomics into routine patient care persist. Realizing the potential of genomics across the clinical care spectrum will require understanding and addressing a range of challenges including

- the costs, availability, accessibility, and coverage of genomic testing;
- the genomic literacy of specialists, primary care providers, and the public;
- the need for clinical decision support tools;
- availability of genetic counselors as well as medical and laboratory geneticists;
- clinical usefulness and actionability of findings;
- the quality, diversity, and broad applicability of reference data sets;
- computing infrastructure capabilities needed to analyze, store, share, and reanalyze vast amounts of genome sequencing data from within and across health care systems; and
- lack of professional guidelines.

[1] The planning committee's role was limited to planning the workshop, and the Proceedings of a Workshop has been prepared by the workshop rapporteurs and listed staff as a factual summary of what occurred at the workshop. Statements, recommendations, and opinions expressed are those of individual presenters and participants, and are not necessarily endorsed or verified by the National Academies of Sciences, Engineering, and Medicine, and they should not be construed as reflecting any group consensus.

1

In 2020, the Roundtable on Genomics and Precision Health of the National Academies of Sciences, Engineering, and Medicine adopted a new strategic plan with the vision of realizing the full potential of health for all through genomics and precision health.[2] This vision moves beyond illness to focus on optimizing health—specifically, how best to integrate genomics into health care practice for the benefit of patients, said Mira Irons, president and CEO of the College of Physicians of Philadelphia.

On October 12, 2022, the roundtable hosted a hybrid public workshop (in Washington, D.C., and via webcast) titled Realizing the Potential of Genomics across the Continuum of Precision Health Care. Greg Feero, professor in the Department of Community and Family Medicine at Geisel School of Medicine and faculty at Maine Dartmouth Family Medicine Residency Program, referred participants to several prior roundtable workshops on related topics including direct-to-consumer genetic testing (IOM and NRC, 2011), the economics of genomic medicine (IOM, 2013), and the adoption of population-scale genomic technology in health systems (NASEM, 2018). The fields of genetics and genomics have advanced, and much has changed in the years since those workshops, he noted. This workshop was intended to spark discussion about how to drive the equitable adoption and implementation of genomics in precision health care,[3] said Michelle Penny, executive vice president of research and development at Embark, Inc. (see Box 1-1 for the workshop planning committee's statement of task).

ORGANIZATION OF THE PROCEEDINGS

This Proceedings of a Workshop summarizes the presentations and discussions that took place during the public workshop held on October 12, 2022.[4] The workshop opened with a keynote presentation on progress made toward the vision of being able to provide a "genome for all who want one" in four key areas: cost, accuracy, speed, and implementation and integration (Chapter 2). In the first session, speakers shared their personal experiences with genetic testing and their perspectives on what patients need as genomics moves into clinical care (Chapter 3). The next session's speakers discussed the concerns of diverse communities and what the speakers noted could

---

[2]The full strategic plan for the Roundtable on Genomics and Precision Health can be found here: https://www.nationalacademies.org/our-work/roundtable-on-genomics-and-precision-health (accessed January 6, 2023).

[3]Genomic data encompass information derived from an individual's DNA, for example, whole genome sequencing data or data from selective panels for pharmacogenomics. The emphasis on clinical sequencing in this workshop proceedings reflects the topics discussed during this workshop.

[4]See the workshop's agenda in Appendix A.

BOX 1-1
Statement of Task

A planning committee of the National Academies of Sciences, Engineering, and Medicine will organize and conduct a public workshop to examine how genomic data are used in health care settings and to identify opportunities for advancement of precision health care delivery. The overarching goal of the workshop is to examine strategies to ensure that genomic applications are responsibly and equitably adopted to benefit populations as well as individuals over time.

The public workshop will feature invited presentations and discussions to explore

- Examples of how genomic data are being used to assess health risk outside of traditional settings for clinical genetics (e.g., prenatal screening and testing, newborn screening, polygenic risk scores) and guide decision making with an eye toward understanding challenges and opportunities related to equity of access to innovation in science and population level adoption of genomic applications;
- How patients, clinicians, and payers assess and act upon the risks and benefits of genomic screening and diagnostic testing; and
- Challenges of integrating genomic data from various sources into clinical decision making including those obtained outside of traditional clinical care settings (e.g., direct-to-consumer, consumer directed, workplace genetic testing) to support equitable precision health care.

The planning committee will organize the workshop, develop the agenda, select and invite speakers and discussants, and moderate or identify moderators for the discussions. A broad array of interested parties may take part in the workshop, including clinicians, genomics experts, users of the health care system (e.g., patients and families), payers, bioethicists, regulators, data scientists, and policy makers. Proceedings of the presentations and discussions at the workshop will be prepared by a designated rapporteur in accordance with institutional guidelines.

help achieve equitable precision care at the health system level (Chapter 4). Speakers then discussed a range of logistical challenges and system-level barriers that need to be addressed for full implementation and integration of genomics in precision health care (Chapters 5 and 6, respectively). The final session (Chapter 7) considered what genomics in health care will look like in the coming decades as well as potential steps to get there and included closing remarks from Christa Martin, chief scientific officer, Geisinger, and professor and director, Autism & Developmental Medical Institute.

2

Improving Health Through Genomics

Highlights of Key Points Made by Euan Ashley

- The aspiration for genomics is to be able to provide a genome "for anyone who wants it...when they want it."
- A genome could be a useful part of an individual's medical record, readily available to warn of the risk for diseases and to inform prescribing by providers.
- The cost of genome sequencing has declined dramatically, accuracy has improved significantly, and speed has increased such that results can be returned within a hospital shift. Much less progress has been made on implementation and integration of genomics into clinical care.
- The application of genomics has expanded far beyond cancer risk screening and diagnosis of rare diseases.
- The diversity of clinical cohorts must be improved so the genetic diversity of the global population is represented.
- Payers need to recognize the health benefits and cost savings of implementing genomics in the delivery of health care.

As a foundation for the workshop, an overview of the increasing use of genomics in precision medicine was provided in a keynote address by Euan Ashley, associate dean of the School of Medicine, Roger and Joelle Burnell Professor of Genomics and Precision Health, and professor of medicine, genetics, biomedical data science, and pathology at Stanford University.[1] A brief discussion followed, moderated by Sarah Wordsworth, professor and university lecturer in the Health Economics Research Centre and Nuffield Department of Population Health at the University of Oxford.

A VISION FOR GENOMICS IN HEALTH CARE

The aspiration for genomics is to be able to provide a genome "for anyone who wants it…when they want it," Ashley said. To achieve the goal of better care through genomics, an individual's genome could be a useful part of their medical record so it is readily available to warn of the risk for thousands of diseases and to inform prescribing by providers. In addition, millions of individual genomes from around the globe could be "seamlessly and securely connected" and linked to a "constantly updated anthology of medical evidence connecting genetic variation and risk of disease," he said.

PROGRESS TOWARD THE GOAL OF BETTER CARE THROUGH GENOMICS

The progress thus far toward realizing the potential of genomics in precision care across the four key areas of cost, accuracy, speed, and implementation and integration was reviewed by Ashley.

Cost

The cost of a high-depth genome over time shows a clear downward trend,[2] which has been compared to the graph for Moore's Law.[3] When sequencing of the human genome was nearing completion, the cost of a complete sequence was roughly $100 million. Decreasing costs tracked with Moore's Law until about 2008, when the cost of sequencing a genome began to drop rapidly until leveling off around 2014, at around $500 per genome, he said. However, in the months before the workshop, several companies announced they would soon be able to offer human genomes for around $100.[4] This trajectory of cost reduction was "unprecedented"

---

[1] See all speakers' full biographies in Appendix B.

[2] For more information on the cost of genome sequencing over time, see https://www.genome.gov/about-genomics/fact-sheets/Sequencing-Human-Genome-cost (accessed January 9, 2023).

[3] Moore's Law, published by Intel cofounder Gordon Moore, predicted the exponential growth of computer processing speed, specifically, that the number of transistors on a microchip would double about every 18 months, while costs would decline (Moore, 1965).

[4] See https://www.science.org/content/article/100-genome-new-dna-sequencers-could-be-game-changer-biology-medicine (accessed February 2, 2023).

in the history of technology and medicine, said Ashley. To illustrate just how striking this reduction in cost is, said Ashley, the cost of a Ferrari 458 Spider in 2013 was about $400,000. If the price of this Ferrari mirrored the price of a human genome, the car would currently cost about 5 cents, and would soon be 1 cent.

While the costs quoted for providing a high-depth genome have dropped dramatically, there are significant capital acquisition costs to be considered for any company or organization entering the field. Some sequencing instruments cost more than $1 million, and some companies do include amortized capital costs into the cost of a genome, Ashley noted. Other factors that affect overall cost include technology, applications, and ancillary costs. The recent expiration of the patent for the sequencing-by-synthesis[5] approach used in clinical sequencing has allowed multiple new companies to enter the field, creating a more competitive pricing environment. Long-read sequencing[6] technologies are becoming available, which are advantageous for accurate germline and somatic sequencing, noted Ashley. These approaches have the potential to illuminate the "dark elements" of the genome that short-read approaches find challenging to assemble.

There are also counting applications (e.g., liquid biopsy, noninvasive prenatal testing) for which short-read sequencing of cell-free DNA or RNA is more cost-effective (cost per gigabase[7] of data). Ancillary costs, including analysis costs and cloud compute costs, have not decreased to the extent that sequencing costs have. Human curation costs have remained steady; however, the time required of a human curator has decreased. Most clinical genomes are currently billed in the range of $3,000 to $12,000, Ashley added. Overall, the progress by the genomics community in reducing the cost of providing a genome deserved a "gold medal," he said.

Accuracy

"Precision medicine needs to be accurate medicine," Ashley said. As discussed, there are limitations to the ability of short-read sequencing to fully characterize the genome, and many of the actionable disease gene variants identified by the American College of Medical Genetics and Genomics were being missed in standard clinical genome sequencing (Ashley, 2016; Dewey et al., 2014). Over the past decade, however, there have been sig-

---

[5]Sequencing by synthesis utilizes fluorescently labeled nucleotides for all four nucleotide bases in DNA to identify the sequence of a piece of DNA as it is being replicated, or synthesized, within tens of millions of clusters parallel. The DNA is sequenced in small reads, typically 300-500 base pairs (Slatko et al., 2018).

[6]Long-read sequencing identifies the sequence from single fragments of DNA in separate wells which allows for reads of 30,000 to 50,000 base pairs (Slatko et al., 2018).

[7]One gigabase equals 1 billion bases (Shchelochkov, 2023).

nificant improvements in the ability to quantify the genome accurately. As examples, Ashley showed the accuracy statistics (F1 scores of 0.9 or higher) from the most recent sequencing challenge hosted by the Genome-in-a-Bottle Consortium of the National Institute of Standards and Technology, and accuracy statistics for three of the top sequencing platforms, noting that, while the technologies each have different strengths, overall accuracy is greatly improved. There are efforts to accurately characterize the full set of more than 6,000 medically relevant genes (Kim et al., 2022). Accuracy is vital for diagnosis; most rare disease genome studies have a diagnosis rate of 30 to 50 percent for previously undiagnosed disease, and most of these findings are actionable (Splinter et al., 2018), Ashley explained. Although the accuracy of genomes has come a long way and continues to improve, there is still more to be done, Ashley said, and he awarded the genomics community a "silver medal" for accuracy.

Speed

The speed of completing a genome has decreased dramatically since the early genomes that took more than 1,000 hours to assemble. In 2012, Kingsmore and colleagues demonstrated the ability to return genomic findings to patients in the neonatal intensive care unit (NICU) in 50 hours (Saunders et al., 2012). In 2014, Ashley and colleagues accomplished the task in 42 hours (Priest et al., 2014). By 2015, Kingsmore had reduced the time needed to 26 hours and was awarded a Guinness World Record for fastest genetic diagnosis (Miller et al., 2015), and in 2018 Kingsmore beat that record with a time of 19.5 hours.[8] Most recently, Ashley and colleagues described returning genomic findings to patients in critical care settings in less than 8 hours, with the most rapid diagnosis made in 7 hours and 20 minutes (Gorzynski et al., 2022). It is likely that the process can be completed even faster, Ashley said. Using the car analogy again to illustrate, Ashley noted that the top speed of the 2013 Ferrari 458 Spider is 199 miles per hour. If the increase in the car's top speed mirrored the increase in speed to deliver genome results the Ferrari would go at 32 million miles per hour. It is now possible to "not just sequence the genome, but return a diagnosis, within one nursing shift," Ashley said, further noting that this is "a major achievement for [the genomics] community" and worthy of a "gold medal."

---

[8]See https://www.rchsd.org/about-us/newsroom/press-releases/new-guinness-world-records-title-set-for-fastest-genetic-diagnosis/ (accessed December 14, 2022).

Implementation and Integration

Working with the technology company SAP, Ashley and colleagues proposed a framework for using natural language processing to integrate genomes and data from wearable sensors into patients' electronic health records (EHRs).[9] As an example, he showed the framework dashboard for a patient in which data from the patient's genome about a cardiac genetic mutation was available together with the patient's diagnosis of cardio-myopathy. While wearable devices have been broadly available to consumers and data have just begun to be integrated into the EHR, the ability to integrate genomes into the EHR and make genomic data accessible is very limited because the genomic data remain largely in PDF form. The EHR provider, Epic, is working to enable the exchange of genetic testing results between laboratories and the Epic system, he noted.

Stanford University has launched an in-house whole-genome sequencing service and provides "a whole-genome backbone for all genetic testing," said Ashley. This allows for *in silico* genetic panels and improved detection of structural variants, he said. Having the full high-depth genome also facilitates the automatic generation of polygenic risk scores. For example, clinical providers will soon be able to easily access a patient's integrated clinical and genomic risk scores for cardiovascular disease. Similarly, pharmacogenomics is beginning to be integrated into the EHR.

A challenge for the integration and implementation of genomics is that diagnostics remain significantly undervalued relative to therapeutics, Ashley said. He observed that the COVID-19 mRNA vaccines were the fastest medicines ever developed, but COVID diagnostics lagged far behind. Another challenge is determining who should pay for genomic diagnostics: health care systems, payers, pharmaceutical companies, or self-pay. Finally, there has been limited integration of genomic data with health care data in the delivery of care.

Overall, Ashley awarded the genomics community a "bronze medal" for efforts thus far to integrate and implement genomics in precision care. There are still challenges to address, particularly regarding inclusion and diversity in clinical genomic research (especially rare disease studies) and the obligations of researchers to study participants who remain undiagnosed when a clinical genomics study concludes (Halley et al., 2022a,b).

GENOMIC MEDICINE: PAST, PRESENT, AND FUTURE

Historically, genomic medicine was limited to cancer applications (genetic testing for inherited risk) and rare diseases (molecular classifica-

---

[9]See https://www.biorxiv.org/content/10.1101/039651v5.full (accessed December 14, 2022).

tion of known disease and undiagnosed disease), Ashley said. The current landscape is much broader and includes early detection and tumor sequencing for cancer; analysis of circulating cell-free DNA for noninvasive prenatal testing, transplant rejection, and liquid biopsy; selective panels for pharmacogenomics; and organism sequencing for infectious diseases. He said the future holds the promise of

- Mendelian, oligogenic, and polygenic architectures for rare diseases;
- circulating cell-free RNA in addition to DNA;
- full comprehensive tumor immunogenomics and detection of minimal residual disease for cancers;
- EHR integration of pharmacogenomic data;
- full microbiome sequencing; and
- integrated polygenic risk scores for common diseases.

"We have come a long way in a short time," Ashley concluded. An individual's genome can now be completed in a matter of hours for the cost of several hundred dollars. Accuracy has improved significantly, owing in part to long-read sequencing, and there are numerous potential near-term applications. However, there is still work to be done to realize the full potential of genomics in precision health care. First, for genomic medicine to be equitable, he said, individuals need to be empowered to obtain their genomic information when they want it, and the diversity of clinical cohorts must be improved so the genetic diversity of the global population is represented. Second, patient-centered planning and decision making could be useful for providing equitable precision health care. Third, genomics could be integrated at the point of care. Finally, payers need to recognize the health benefits and cost savings of implementing genomics in the delivery of health care, he said.

DISCUSSION

"The genome is not one size fits all," said a workshop participant, noting that while the information gleaned from the genome may be useful for different purposes across the life span, everyone does not necessarily need genome sequencing right now. Perhaps, the participant suggested, the focus should be on when genome sequencing is needed and figuring out how to implement it. From a public health perspective, Ashley said, the right approach is probably a stepwise approach where what could be done is thought about first as well as who would get the most benefit. Taking a system perspective, he further clarified that if the field's responsibility is to do the most good, it should work from there to something aspirational like a genome for everyone who wants it to empower those who want to have access to this type of health information.

David Ledbetter, chief clinical and research officer at Unified Patient Network, Inc. and professor in the department of psychiatry at the University of Florida, commented that the United Kingdom (UK) seems to be well ahead of the United States on the implementation of genomics in clinical care. For example, the UK recently announced the launch of a 5-million-person polygenic risk score clinical study.[10] The UK is at the forefront of clinical genomics, and this is attributable in part to the fact that the UK has a single-payer system, Ashley suggested. Having a national health service allows for the uptake of genomics rapidly and at scale. The UK's progress in implementing genomics also stems from the efforts of individuals who have championed genomics, whether at the grassroots level, in political or governmental leadership, or leaders of the medical community, he added.

In response to a workshop participant's question, Ashley said that even as genomic technology advances, the patient's personal family medical history will always remain very important across all aspects of care. A genome can help clarify elements of family history that are forgotten or not known and better empower patients to understand risk.

---

[10]https://www.genomeweb.com/microarrays-multiplexing/uk-researchers-aim-discern-new-polygenic-risk-scores-5-million-genotypes#.Y63ndnbMI2w (accessed December 29, 2022).

3

Enabling Patients to Benefit from Genomics

Highlights of Key Points Made by Individual Speakers

- Patients and families would benefit from receiving relevant or actionable information about genetic testing for markers that can predict disease risk at an early stage. (Goto, Henley, Norris)
- Engaging with communities using approaches that are culturally competent and at the appropriate literacy level could help raise awareness of the potential benefits of genetic testing. (Henley)
- Equitable access to genomics and precision medicine could be improved by addressing the many factors that affect access such as having a health care provider, costs and coverage, transportations challenges, language barriers, cultural barriers, health literacy, the informed consent process, bias, and racism. (Norris)
- Improve the care pathway so the interpretation, counseling, and care plan a patient receives after genetic testing are not affected by the clinical providers they see and the testing product that is used. (Radford)
- Earlier diagnosis of rare diseases can improve outcomes for patients and their families; therefore, clinicians may benefit from training in identifying patients who could benefit from genomic screening tools. (Goto)

- Centralized services and resources for genetic and rare disorders, including testing, genetic counselors, and care coordinators, could be helpful in rural areas. (Goto)
- Research, education, and training in genetic and rare disorders may be essential, including workforce development, care services mapping, support for access to patient registries and clinical trials, and the development of virtual specialty clinics. (Goto)

NOTE: This list is the rapporteurs' summary of points made by the individual speakers identified, and the statements have not been endorsed or verified by the National Academies of Sciences, Engineering, and Medicine. They are not intended to reflect a consensus among workshop participants.

"[Genomic] screening is a tool that should be used to identify and prevent diseases sooner," said Candace Henley, founder and chief surviving officer of the Blue Hat Foundation and session comoderator. "Underserved and intentionally marginalized communities have higher rates of late-stage diseases, disability, and death," she said, and the lack of information about disease risk is a contributing factor. People in these communities are missing opportunities to be proactively screened for disease risk and to take preventive action based on family history.

To set the stage for the discussion, Henley shared her personal story of being diagnosed with colorectal cancer in 2003 at age 35. The pathology report noted microsatellite instability and she was told she had Lynch syndrome. She was given no information, no one asked about her family history, and genetic testing was never discussed. Henley said she was not aware of the hereditary nature of her cancer and that it was something she should make her children and family members aware of. Even at subsequent visits with her physician there was no discussion of family history. Years later, Henley found out that autopsies done after the deaths of her father and two aunts revealed that they each had colon cancer at the time they died. None of them knew they had the disease, and the autopsy findings were not shared with the family, she said.

Patient access to actionable information about genetic testing is still lacking today, Henley said, and many physicians are not trained to talk about genetic testing. Further, genetic counselors are not recognized as health care providers by the Centers for Medicare & Medicaid Services (CMS), leaving those covered by Medicaid or Medicare to rely on their physician to recommend and interpret genetic testing. Many people who would benefit from genetic testing are not aware of what genetic testing is or its importance, so Henley said it can be useful to raise community awareness through approaches that are culturally competent and at the appropriate literacy level. A patient who appears indifferent when receiving medical information might, in fact, be afraid to ask questions, she added. Henley encouraged providers to avoid implicit bias and make sure that patients understand the information being shared by asking them to report back what they heard.

Instead of asking patients to implicitly trust the system, "the system has to become trustworthy for patients," and one of the ways systems can do this is to "trust the patients who are in front of them" instead of making assumptions, added Gwen Darien, executive vice president for patient advocacy and engagement at the National Patient Advocate Foundation and session comoderator.

In this panel session, speakers shared their personal experiences with genetic testing, and their perspectives on what patients need as genomics moves into clinical care.

EQUITABLE PRECISION MEDICINE

Keri Norris, vice president of health equity, diversity, and inclusion at the National Hemophilia Foundation, described rushing to the intensive care unit of a hospital several states away to be at the bedside of her 31-year old son during the COVID-19 pandemic. He had been admitted through the emergency department where they found his heart ejection fraction was 10 percent. Her son was a healthy, active young adult who had never been hospitalized and had only had a minor surgery as a young child, she said. After several months she was able to have him transferred to a hospital near her in Atlanta, Georgia, where doctors decided to order genetic tests. Norris said the tests identified "two markers that could have easily predicted that this was going to happen at some point in time in his life." Had the family had that information earlier, her son would likely not be in need of a heart transplant today, she said.

Communities and families need information about genetic markers that can predict disease risk at an early stage, but many are not aware of screening or do not know where to get it, Norris said, echoing Henley. Genetic risk information is useful for all people, regardless of their economic status, where they live, or their insurance status, she said. She called upon health care professionals to advocate for equitable precision medicine. Having access to precision medicine goes beyond just having insurance coverage and a primary care physician, Norris said. There are multiple other considerations that need to be supported, such as interactions with clinical providers; the ability to get to appointments, to balance competing interests, and to get information about genetic testing; and knowing or being taught how to use that information, Norris pointed out. She highlighted several areas for attention.

- **Transportation.** Many patients face transportation challenges getting to and from routine clinical visits and specialist visits. The need to meet with genetic counselors, a clinical research team, or other genomic medical professionals adds to that challenge, Norris noted. Solutions are needed to ensure that once patients are informed about genetic testing, they can make it to their appointments, she added.
- **Cost.** Even if a genome will only cost $100, "That's a stretch for the average American," Norris said. Genetic testing and genomic medicine should not be only for those with the ability to pay, she added. Costs—and who covers those costs—are considerations.
- **Relationships.** Consider whether the patient has a relationship with a primary care physician that has access to genetic tests, as well as what the relationship of the payer is, Norris said.
- **Language and translation services.** Information about genomics and precision medicine would be useful if it were effectively and efficiently available to patients regardless of whether English is their primary language, she said.
- **Cultural considerations.** It is also important to consider how practices in genomics and precision medicine mesh with, and might translate into, the diverse cultures of patients, their families, and their communities, Norris said.
- **Health literacy.** Information and instructions concerning genetic testing and study participation could be meaningful, written in plain language, and easy for patients to understand, Norris said.
- **Informed consent.** When patients agree to participate in clinical research in genetics, including gene therapy studies, it is important that they fully understand what they are consenting to, including the inclusion and exclusion criteria. It may be essential that they understand that they can withdraw from the study.
- **Bias.** Implicit or unconscious bias among medical professionals leads to assumptions about patients that can affect how providers interact with patients and the information or medical treatment the patients receive. These biases can result in providers not even asking certain populations if they want genetic testing, she said. Experiencing bias can also result in patients not returning to a provider for continued care. Norris reflected on her experience where assumptions were made when she arrived at the hospital as the patient's mother in casual dress, and she was treated differently versus when she is seen as Dr. Norris, a recognized public health professional. She experienced blatant bias toward her son from some of the clinical providers.
- **Racism in medicine.** "We need to recognize that racism is real in medicine and work towards dismantling it," Norris said. She

described personally experiencing racism in health care on "multiple occasions over the past year." Since her son was young, assumptions were made that his heart condition must be attributable to lifestyle and behavior choices, she said. "No one thought about genetics. ... They just went straight to blaming the patient," she said.

DIAGNOSING RARE DISEASES

Ayanna's Story

Greta Goto, founding member of the Prader-Willi Syndrome (PWS) Alaska Parent Group, and cochair of the Community Engagement in Genomics Working Group of the National Human Genome Research Institute, shared her experiences with genetic testing and care as the parent of a daughter with a rare disease.

Goto's daughter, Ayanna, was born in Anchorage and despite having "a very weak cry, was floppy, did not suck, [and] had a poor appetite," Goto said that they were discharged 10 days later to their home in Dillingham without a diagnosis after various tests were inconclusive. Over the next 4 years she missed all the usual development milestones, and since there are no specialists in the small town of Dillingham, the family had to regularly bring Ayanna to specialists in Anchorage, which Goto noted is 339 air miles from Dillingham and cost $450–600 round trip per person at that time. They continued this diagnostic odyssey until Ayanna was finally diagnosed in 1997 at age 4.5 after a friend of a friend had a son with PWS who had similar symptoms and behaviors as Ayanna, Goto said. Alaska's rural health clinic in Dillingham connected Goto with the traveling genetics clinic from Seattle Children's Hospital in Washington, and a specialist was able to see Ayanna in Dillingham. Genetic testing confirmed Ayanna had PWS, "a rare disease affecting 1 in 15,000 to 20,000 people," Goto said. There is no cure for PWS and people with it "are always going to need help."

During her middle school and high school years Ayanna faced increasing, serious challenges and "she needed mental health interventions, behavioral health interventions, medication management, and continued individualized education plan support," Goto said. Applying for a Medicaid waiver for supports for a person with disabilities is complicated, laborious, and often overwhelming, including being placed on a wait list which is a process that is repeated yearly, Goto explained. Goto described how, at age 22, Ayanna and her family faced more transitions in securing funding to support the services and trained staff she continued to need. This "disability cliff"[1] included

---

[1] The disability cliff is the loss of federal entitlement to special education of individuals with disabilities, generally at age 22 (Bagenstos, 2015).

extensive additional administrative tasks. Ayanna is now 29 years old, and her parents and caregivers are working hard to secure her care and safety for the long term. Many medical and education professionals do not understand the complexities of managing the care of someone with PWS, Goto added.

Goto said she and her husband often wonder if Ayanna's situation might be different if she had been diagnosed as an infant and had timely access to the best practices for PWS patients (e.g., growth hormone therapy). Although this is not the life they had envisioned for Ayanna when she was born, they have worked hard to "help her help herself." Ayanna graduated from high school, loves art and dancing, volunteers, and hopes to have a job. She is also a "super voter" and looks at whether candidates support disability services as well as the people who work in disability services. She has learned to advocate for herself, such as telling providers they can talk directly to her, instead of to her mother about her, she said.

Challenges in Underresourced Areas

Despite the speed with which genome sequencing can now be done, the average time to get a rare disease diagnosis in the United States is still 6 to 7 years. Earlier diagnosis is needed to improve outcomes for patients and their families, Goto said. Services and resources for genetic and rare disorders are scarce, particularly in rural regions. In Alaska, there are few resources outside of the urban hubs along the "Railbelt" (which is "the only part of Alaska where you can drive from community to community," Goto said). Alaska has very few genetics counselors, a shortage of care coordinators, no medical school, and services are often provided by genetics professionals who travel from the lower 48 states. Finding in-state support systems is difficult, as is accessing services and supports outside of Alaska, Goto said. Further, she has "little confidence in health insurance providers understanding the complexity of a genetic disorder and needs for ongoing care." Ultimately, the parents become the experts in their child's disorder, she added. "We have to tell medical professionals what to do and what to be looking for, and yet we are not respected as a part of the care team," Goto said. Parents and extended family who provide care experience burnout, and the siblings of the affected child also need support.

Although her observations are specific to her family's experiences in Alaska, others across the country face similar challenges, particularly those in rural areas and in U.S. territories, which she said should not be forgotten.

Improving Access to Genetic Care and Resources

Goto closed with several suggestions for improving access and availability of genetic and rare disorder care resources in her state of Alaska that she said would be of great help to families. Centralized services with testing, counseling, and other resources could be helpful, and statistics could be collected on rates of genetic and rare disorders in the state, she noted. A needs assessment could be done of the known rare disorder population and their caregivers to identify how to better serve patients after diagnosis, Goto added. Best practices for integrated care coordination could be identified and deployed that bring together the services and supports needed to address both medical and social needs for people with genetic and rare disorders and their caregivers, Goto said. Research, education, and training in genetic and rare disorders may be essential, including workforce development, care services mapping, support for access to patient registries and clinical trials, and the development of virtual specialty clinics. Finally, Goto said advocacy, partnerships, and fundraising could help to support genetic and rare disorder care.

THE CARE NAVIGATION MAZE

Cristi Radford, product director at Optum, described her personal diagnostic journey from her unique perspective as a certified genetic counselor who has spent her career in the development and implementation of genetics products and services. Her family history of cancer also had an effect on her journey. Radford's mother, who had a family history of breast and prostate cancer, was diagnosed with a brain tumor in her thirties and melanoma in her sixties. Radford's brother developed melanoma in his thirties. "I don't think any of us would be surprised to find an inherited cancer gene mutation in this family," she said.

Receiving Unexpected Results

In late 2018, while working on a direct-to-consumer genome product, Radford decided to send her own sample out for testing "to get the patient experience for the product." Although possible that her results could show an increased risk for cancer, she knew it was unlikely as her family had previously had basic genetic testing. Based on these previous genetic tests and family history, the most likely risk that would show up would be for genes associated with skin cancers, which she already knew she had an increased risk for. In April of 2019, Radford received a 153-page report with some of the expected results, as well as the very unexpected result of potential increased risk for multiple endocrine neoplasia (MEN), which includes a risk for an aggressive type of thyroid cancer. Confirmatory testing was needed, Radford said, and she ordered a large inherited cancer panel because, in addition to her family history, she also had a palpable breast lump and was undergoing evaluation to rule out breast cancer.

Because of her career and her network, she had a level of access that others do not, Radford pointed out.

Unable to get an endocrinology appointment at Moffitt Cancer Center for 3 months, Radford tried to understand her actual risk of MEN from terms in the initial and confirmatory reports such as "potential lower penetrance" and "mild phenotype" and "95 percent risk" and called around to different laboratories to get a better understanding of the risk assessments. She also did not want to wait until the appointment at Moffitt to have her calcitonin level tested (high levels can indicate thyroid cancer) and found that individuals can order this test themselves at Quest Direct for $60. She said she considered $60 a minimal cost to find out quickly that she likely did not have metastatic disease at that moment.

Two months later, Radford was able to discuss her case with an endocrinologist at MD Anderson and then shortly thereafter had her appointment with the endocrinologists at Moffitt. She noted that a colleague who was an academic genetic counselor attended these appointments with her virtually. Based on her mutation and the associated risk, the endocrinologists recommended against removing Radford's thyroid because many people who have thyroids removed do not return to "normal." Instead, they recommended a care plan including periodic screening with blood tests and thyroid ultrasound.

A Resource-Intensive Journey

It was an eye-opener to discover how much time is needed to define a path forward after receiving genetic results that indicate increased risk of disease, Radford said. Because of her career she has easy access to services, resources, and experts, and yet it took nearly 7 months before she had a comprehensive care plan and baseline screenings complete, she reiterated.

In addition to the chronological time span, Radford used seven paid time off (PTO) days during that first year for endocrine, breast, and skin exam appointments. She was able to coordinate visits with specialists during business trips so she did not lose extra PTO to travel. Adding on the 2.5 days used for her usual well visits (primary care, gynecology, dental, vision) made a total of nearly 10 PTO days used for health appointments that year with risk for just one main cancer, yet some people have increased risk for multiple cancers. According to the Bureau of Labor and Statistics, the average PTO allowance for private-sector employees with a year of service is 10 days (Spencer, 2019). People also need time off for other obligations and personal plans (e.g., medical appointments for children and family members, family obligations, sick children), she added. "We're asking them to use all of their time off to develop a screening plan, and then we wonder, why do people have gaps in care? This is not realistic," Radford said.

There are also financial effects of surveillance. Radford said the associated medical costs of establishing her care plan were about $3,000, and she estimated that out-of-pocket costs going forward would be about $1,700 per screen. Her out-of-pocket costs for 2022 in June were nearly $3,000, and she anticipated this would increase because of the necessary follow-up appointments. For a person earning $45,000 per year, $3,000 represents more than 6 percent of their annual income. "How is the average American supposed to do this?" Radford asked.

Radford also described her brother's journey to illustrate that the counseling and care plan one gets depends on the providers they see. Because of their family history of cancer, her brother had done preconception carrier screening in 2016 through a commercial laboratory. He was seen by a genetic counselor employed by the laboratory who only discussed their product, Radford pointed out. At that time a larger cancer panel was not done despite being informed of a family history of cancer. Later, after Radford received her genomic results, her brother also underwent genome sequencing. He saw a different genetic counselor who did not have a background in cancer, resulting in many unanswered questions, anxiety, and urgent care visits, she added. Ultimately, his care plan recommended thyroid surgery. After the surgery, his thyroid was found to be normal, and he has struggled to find the right balance of thyroid medication, she reported. In retrospect, Radford wondered how having a larger cancer panel done in 2016 might have affected or better informed her brother's choices when conceiving children.

The goal of genomic testing is to improve health outcomes, Radford said. There is a lot of focus on the "diagnostic odyssey"—who needs to be tested, access to testing, and test selection. However, attention could be aimed at examining what happens after people receive their report, including clinician interpretation, development of a care plan, and delivery of follow-up services. Care navigation can be a maze, and new pathways could be useful as genomes become more broadly accessible. "These need to be supported by laboratories, insurers, clinicians, and employers if we really want to improve health outcomes," she concluded.

DISCUSSION

Investing in Both Technology and Practice

"Genomic technology is a tool," and could be used in a way that aligns with patient preferences and helps them to achieve their health goals, moderator Darien said. It would be helpful for the medical establishment to decide what it is trying to accomplish with genomic tools, and how those goals might differ if the tools are used for diagnosis versus proactive assessment of potential disease risk, Radford said. She received a very unexpected genomic result from a direct-to-consumer genome product and "Now I'm dealing with this for the rest of my life." Decisions about continuing screening and incurring the financial and time costs versus not doing anything and accepting the risk versus removing a healthy thyroid is now something Radford has to consider. In Darien's 25 years working in patient advocacy, a key issue for many women with cancer is whether the results of testing will be actionable and how the findings will affect their lives, she said.

More investment could be useful in both developing genomic tools and improving the ability of practitioners to identify those who could benefit from these tools, Goto said. She shared an example of this from an individual whose newborn had signs of PWS at birth, but as there was no genetic counselor on staff at the hospital, the baby was subject to a series of unnecessary tests and procedures. Investment in access to resources for patients after they are diagnosed with a genetic disorder is also needed, she said, recalling their struggle to get services and resources after Ayanna's diagnosis. In addition to genetic counseling, Henley said that mental health counseling could also be available to people when they receive genomic results as the information received is often unexpected and can be distressing.

Promoting Equity and Addressing Bias

A theme throughout the panel presentations was patients feeling that they were not being seen or heard and that providers were making assumptions influenced by implicit biases instead of getting to know the patient and their needs, Darien summarized. Panelists continued the discussion of bias and racism in medicine and how implicit bias in the practice of clinical genomics could be addressed.

Henley shared that her brother passed away in 2020 after experiencing rectal bleeding for 6 years. He had a fear of hospitals and was also very afraid of learning whether he had cancer like she had, and so he "self-medicated by drinking," she said. When he did go to the emergency room, they would start by giving him Tylenol and then, because he would leave out of fear, he was labeled as drug seeking. Henley advocated for him, emphasizing that they would not have come to the emergency room if he only needed Tylenol. He was finally diagnosed with hemophilia. Health care providers needed to "stop looking at the fact that he's a Black man and look at the fact that he is a person in need of medical care" and "view him as a loving, viable human being that has loved ones waiting on him to return home," she said. Stop blaming the patient for what is a failing of the health care system to meet their needs, Henley said.

Norris said that the first step to overcoming implicit bias is self-awareness, which is then followed by self-regulation. Creating self-awareness takes more than one training session. Education about unconscious bias and the need for cultural humility needs to start early, as part of medical school curriculums, and it needs to be embedded into clinical practice (e.g., required training modules), she said. It is also important to listen to patients when they call with concerns about their care experiences, or when surveys suggest that patients from minoritized and marginalized populations are having poor experiences with certain providers, and then take steps to address the issues, Norris said. Henley suggested that providers can put their bias training to work by doing community engagement or volunteering with community organizations to bring information to the community.

Avoid the pitfalls of continuing to work in silos on issues of health equity, Norris emphasized. Bring all parties to the table when developing toolkits, resources, and guidelines and recommendations, Norris suggested. Take the time to reach out to communities, listen, and understand their needs. She noted that the challenges of addressing the social determinants of health can appear overwhelming. However, "Victory comes in inches, not miles, and we have to start today working together to ensure equitable outcomes and health for all," she said.

4

Building an Equitable Precision Health Care System

Highlights of Key Points Made by Individual Speakers

- Social determinants of health and population demographics need to be considered when researching and implementing genomics and precision medicine tools; otherwise, existing health disparities will be further exacerbated. (Baker)
- Mistrust of the medical establishment stems from historical and ongoing mistreatment of racial, minoritized groups and other underrepresented populations. The onus is on the medical establishment to become trustworthy, and clinicians and researchers can work together with their communities to build and maintain trust. (Baker, Wilkins)
- Develop clinical and research workforces that are diverse and representative of the populations they serve and provide continuing education and resources for professionals on working with diverse patient populations. (Baker, Wilkins)
- Funding is needed to close the large gaps in quality reference data for diverse populations; persons of non-European descent are significantly underrepresented in genome-wide association studies, and the benefits of treatments and tools developed based on these studies do not translate equally to all people. (Wilkins)
- Embedding genomic testing in institutional policies that direct best practices in care reduces provider-based variability.

Genomic testing then becomes routine for all patients, regardless of background, sex, race, or ancestry. (Relling)

NOTE: This list is the rapporteurs' summary of points made by the individual speakers identified, and the statements have not been endorsed or verified by the National Academies of Sciences, Engineering, and Medicine. They are not intended to reflect a consensus among workshop participants.

Building on the personal perspectives of equity in genomic medicine that were shared by the first panel, the second session speakers discussed the concerns of diverse communities and what can be done to help achieve equitable precision care at the health system level. The session was moderated by Gabriel Lázaro-Muñoz, assistant professor of psychiatry and member of the Harvard Medical School Center for Bioethics at Harvard Medical School.

ADDRESSING THE NEEDS AND CONCERNS OF DIVERSE COMMUNITIES

A Focus on Sexual and Gender Minorities

"For precision medicine to be successful, we need to make sure that we are thinking about it not just in the clinic, but also from the perspective of the social determinants of health, the things that happen outside of the clinical setting that really affect how well our medical technologies and our treatments work," said Kellan Baker, executive director and chief learning officer at the Whitman-Walker Institute. Not taking social determinants of health—as well as patient demographics such as race, ethnicity, disability, sexual orientation, and gender—into account when implementing precision medicine tools and technologies will exacerbate existing disparities and further disadvantage already underserved populations, he said.

Barriers to the Uptake of Genomics and Precision Care

To benefit from precision medicine, patients must have access to it, Baker said. Some of the barriers to access that can disproportionately affect diverse and underserved populations include costs of care, insurance coverage of evaluations and treatments, availability of providers with expertise in precision medicine, and transportation to the provider's office, Baker said. Health literacy also affects access, and Baker noted that information about the availability and benefits of new medical breakthroughs often does not reach diverse populations, especially those who do not receive routine clinical care. Discrimination also affects access to precision medicine, both directly, and because "Previous and anticipated experiences of discrimination in health care settings create medical mistrust," Baker said.

Many individuals and communities are skeptical about advances, such as within precision medicine, and harbor concerns that they could be hurt, or that they will once again give of themselves and receive nothing in return. For example, there is great mistrust of genomic research and precision medicine among many lesbian, gay, bisexual, transgender, and queer (LGBTQ) persons, Baker noted. This stems from a history of mistreatment of LGBTQ individuals in medical care: a recent nationwide study showed that LGBTQ respondents were more than three times as likely than non-LGBTQ individuals to "postpone or avoid getting medical care because they were afraid of mistreatment," Baker said. LGBTQ patients may also mistrust genomics because of misguided research efforts to identify a so-called "gay gene" or a "trans gene," which raise concerns of eugenics should such genes ever be found, he added.

Making Genomics and Precision Medicine Acceptable to Patients

"Medical mistrust is not a condition to be cured of," Baker said. "It is an adaptive response to historical and ongoing mistreatment." The onus is on the medical establishment to become trustworthy. One approach is to develop a workforce that better reflects the communities it serves, meaning patients are served by clinicians and researchers who have similar racial or other backgrounds. This requires creating career paths that attract and retain people of color, women, people with disabilities, and people who identify as LGBTQ, Baker said. Evidence suggests that these populations drop out of science, technology, engineering, and math (STEM) and health career pathways early on. For example, it is estimated that the representation of LGBTQ people in STEM fields is 20 percent less than expected, he said. Often when students do not see health or research professionals who look like them, they have difficulty envisioning themselves in those roles.

Another approach is to ensure that clinicians and researchers receive continuing education, training, and resources on working with diverse populations. Baker observed that there is much attention on advancing the technical aspects of science and medicine, but these tools can be of limited use if they are not implemented or administered. Genomic medicine tools must be acceptable to, and understandable by, patients and broader communities, and trainings as well as other resources that incorporate the experiences and concerns of diverse patient populations need to be readily available to, and taken up by, clinicians and researchers, he said. For example, Baker said that resources for working effectively with LGBTQ patients exist but are often viewed as difficult to find.

Incorporating Patient Identities and Experiences

Precision medicine's focus on the genome and specific therapeutic targets mean that the focus on the person at the center of this approach can be lost, Baker observed. Data on people's identities and day-to-day experiences could help inform the effective use of these advances, he added. The field is lacking data on patient sex, gender identity, and sexual orientation; precise definitions of what is meant by these terms; and methods for how best to collect these data. In 2022, a consensus study committee at the National Academies of Sciences, Engineering, and Medicine[1] released recommended standards for the collection of data on sex, gender identity, and sexual orientation, Baker noted (NASEM, 2022). These are all "complex multidimensional elements of human identity" that are being incorrectly broken down into a simple binary, he said. For example, sex includes components of genetics, anatomy, and hormones, and one's sex as assigned on a birth certificate dictates how a child is raised and the way the world interacts with them but may not reflect the individual's true gender. Baker asked, "Does the truth of who we are really lie in our genes, or is it instead a really complex relationship between the genome [and] so many other elements of our biology, of our surroundings, of our upbringings?"

A Focus on Racial and Ethnic Minority Groups

Health equity is "the absence of avoidable, unfair, or remediable differences in health outcomes among socially disadvantaged populations,"[2] said Consuelo Wilkins, chief equity officer, professor of medicine, senior vice president, and senior associate dean for Health Equity and Inclusive Excellence, and engagement core director for the All of Us research program at Vanderbilt University Medical Center. "Precision medicine has been built on a foundation of inequity," she said. Inequitable practices in health care, precision medicine, and genomics have resulted in flawed science. Nearly 80 percent of the individuals in the genome-wide association studies (GWAS) catalog are of European ancestry. Although inclusion of non-European ancestry individuals in GWAS has increased over the last decade, they are still woefully underrepresented (Popejoy and Fullerton, 2016; Quansah and McGregor, 2017; Sirugo et al., 2019). As such, the benefits of the treatments and tools, such as diagnostics, screening tests, and algorithms, that were developed based on these studies do not translate equally to all people, she said. The population of the world continues to change, and 80 percent of the global population is expected to be of Asian

---

[1]Herein referred to as "the National Academies."

[2]Adapted from the World Health Organization. See https://www.who.int/health-topics/social-determinants-of-health#tab=tab_3 (accessed December 14, 2022).

or African descent by 2050, Wilkins added. Therefore, reference data sets need to change, she emphasized.

Race, Ethnicity, and Genetic Testing

"Race is a sociopolitical construct," Wilkins said. Although there can be some overlap with ancestry, people are grouped into races based on physical characteristics, and race-based discrimination and oppression persist in the United States. Although there is no biological basis for race, it cannot be disassociated from health, Wilkins said.

There is much discussion of how to use race in science going forward, whether or how genetic ancestry might be used in place of race, and how categorizing people affects genomics and precision health (Lewis et al., 2022). Wilkins discussed research being done by the Vanderbilt-Miami-Meharry Precision Medicine Disparities Collaborative using samples from Vanderbilt's DNA biorepository which are linked to medical records. This research found that when race is controlled for, the disorders that are most associated with African genetic ancestry, determined by GWAS, are kidney disease and sickle cell anemia. However, when instead of race, genetic ancestry is controlled for, the conditions most associated with those who identify by race as Black or African American are hypertension and fatigue, conditions that are often associated with allostatic load and with one's environment (e.g., experiencing racism and discrimination, living in disinvested communities), Wilkins said.

Current genetic screening and diagnostic tests do not provide equal benefit for all populations, Wilkins said. Studies have shown that rates of variants of uncertain or unknown significance (VUSs) are higher in racial or ethnic minority individuals compared to individuals of European ancestry (Kwon et al., 2020; Ndugga-Kabuye and Issaka, 2019; Roberts et al., 2020). Yet, there are few discussions of revisiting these VUSs to determine their significance, she said.

Improving Equity in Precision Health Care

In general, the delivery of health care is inequitable, and this is not unique to genomics and precision medicine. The blame is often placed on implicit bias, but Wilkins said there is evidence that the root cause of racial and ethnic disparities in health care is racism (IOM, 2003), adding:

> If we don't actually take steps to try to dismantle the systemic and structural racism that continues to enable these systems to exclude people, then we're really not addressing the root causes [of inequitable care].

Further, many of the inequities in health outcomes could be attributable not to genetics, but to the body's response to the physiological stress of conditions such as living in poverty or in a disinvested community, experiencing racism, or having an increased allostatic load, she suggested. These stressors "are increasing [the] risk of disease, including risk of epigenetic changes that could lead to disease," Wilkins said (Carlos et al., 2022). "We can talk about access. We can talk about all sorts of things. But if we're not going to address the underlying racism, then we're not going to get very far," she added.

Wilkins concluded her talk by highlighting opportunities for building equitable precision health care:

- Committing funding to closing the large gap in quality reference data for diverse populations. These new data could identify novel genomic variants, establish clinical relevance, and interpret VUSs. Incremental steps will not close the data gap; a large injection of funding to support increased activity is needed.
- Acknowledging that some racial and ethnic groups are benefiting less from precision medicine and precision health and committing to remedying that.
- Recognizing that delivering on the promise of precision medicine involves more than genetics and genomics and incorporating information on patients' social and structural determinants of health in precision health care.
- Increasing diversity in the health care and research workforce, and reaching out to, and engaging with, marginalized communities.
- Understanding and incorporating the needs and priorities of minority groups in precision health care by involving communities in study design.
- Working to build trust in health care and clinical research. "Acknowledge again that people have real reasons to distrust us based on our past and current activities and the way we deliver care and provide and perform research," she concluded.

CASE EXAMPLE:
REDUCING BIAS BY IMPLEMENTING PANEL-BASED PREEMPTIVE PHARMACOGENETIC TESTING FOR EVERYONE

"Most adults and many children receive at least one high-risk actionable pharmacogenetic drug in their lifetime,"[3] said Mary Relling, coinvestigator

---

[3] An example of a high-risk actionable pharmacogenetic drug is clopidogrel or warfarin (Schildcrout et al., 2012).

and cofounder of the Clinical Pharmacogenetics Implementation Consortium (CPIC)[4] and member of the Pharmaceutical Sciences Department at St. Jude Children's Research Hospital (Chan et al., 2021; Chanfreau-Coffinier et al., 2019; Kimpton et al., 2019; Kuch et al., 2016; Samwald et al., 2016). In addition, more than 95 percent of the U.S. population has a high-risk diplotype for at least one of the original 12 genes identified by CPIC as pharmacogenetically actionable (Dunnenberger et al., 2015).

In any given year, about half of the patients at St. Jude Children's Research Hospital will receive at least one high-risk drug, Relling said. The cost of multigene panel testing is comparable to that of single gene testing and so, in 2011, St. Jude Children's Research Hospital launched the PG4KDS protocol to implement panel-based preemptive pharmacogenetic testing as the standard of care for all consenting patients (Haidar et al., 2022).[5] This approach supports the mission of St. Jude to "advance cures, and means of prevention, for pediatric catastrophic diseases through research and treatment," as well as the hospital's culture of evidence-based prescribing, she said.

Implementing the PG4KDS Protocol

Pharmacogenetic Testing in Children

St. Jude Children's Research Hospital believes "There is no ethical reason to exclude children from preemptive pharmacogenetic testing," Relling said. Germline genomic variants do not change as a person ages, and CPIC gene–drug prescribing guidelines are applicable to children. She highlighted some of the special considerations for pharmacogenomic testing in pediatric patients at St. Jude. Parents provide consent on behalf of underage patients, which includes specific consent for the possibility of finding sex chromosome abnormalities. Consent is obtained again directly from the patient when they reach 18 years of age, and Relling noted that most pediatric practices have patients who have reached adulthood. At St. Jude, "Parents are not allowed to refuse incidental findings on behalf of their child," Relling said. The incidental findings that must be reported to parents and patients are those that have "a very strong association with disease risk, [are] not likely to be discovered via other means, and [are] actionable before the child reaches 18 years of age," she explained.

---

[4]CPIC was established in 2009 to "create, curate, update, [and] make freely available specific peer-reviewed, evidence-based, updatable clinical guidelines for actionable gene/drug pairs," Relling said. See https://cpicpgx.org (accessed December 14, 2022).

[5]See also www.stjude.org/pg4kds/implement (accessed December 14, 2022).

The Process

The PG4KDS process begins with research nurses identifying patients for potential enrollment in the protocol from the daily list of new patients, and Relling said that nearly all are approached to participate (Hoffman et al., 2014). Of patients that are asked, more than 95 percent consent to participate and more than 96 percent of participants reconsent at age 18. Pharmacogenetic testing to inform prescribing is considered to be part of the patient's medical care, "similar to how we would treat administration of flu vaccine," Relling said. Testing is approved by an oversight committee, implemented institution-wide, and each enrollment in the protocol does not require consultation with the primary physician. Once enrolled, a blood sample is collected and more than 1,100 genes are genotyped. All results are entered into the research database, and results for select genes are entered into the patient's electronic health record (those for which there is clinical decision support available for at least one drug affected by the gene), she explained.

Because genomic findings have life-long implications, genotype results are entered into a dedicated pharmacogenetics tab in the EHR so they are not encounter specific, Relling explained. The EHR contains the diplotype, the interpretation, and patient letter and is uploaded to the patient portal. High-risk diplotypes are also automatically populated into the patient's problem list as phenotypes and are linked to clinical decision support that guides prescribing through interruptive alerts, she said. There are also pretest alerts that are triggered for select gene–drug pairs when the relevant genetic test result is absent from the patient record. Clinical decision support grows more complex when more than one gene affects prescribing for a drug, Relling said. Standardization of terminology is important for sharing data across EHR systems, she noted.

Progress

More than 6,600 patients have been enrolled in PG4KDS and genotyped, and around 53 percent are White, Relling said. Thus far the protocol has been implemented for 14 genes that affect a total of 66 drugs, and 95 percent of patients at St. Jude have been found to have at least one high-risk phenotype for those 14 genes. Adherence to the prescribing advice in the clinical decision support alerts among practitioners has been very high (92 percent) over the past decade (Nguyen et al., 2022).

Relling reviewed the process for implementing a new gene–drug pair beginning with results interpretation, clinical consultations, creation of problem list entries, and development of clinical decision support, which is done using the resources of CPIC. This is a time-consuming process, and only one or two new genes are added per year. St. Jude then updates its formulary, drug policies, patient and provider educational materials, and clinical competencies; approval is obtained from the pharmacogenetics oversight committee; and information about the new gene–drug pair is shared publicly, she said.

The expansion of precision medicine, including clinical genomics and pharmacogenomic testing, is now part of the St. Jude Children's Research Hospital strategic plan and is supported by institutional leadership, Relling said. Pharmacogenomic testing for thiopurines is also now an institutional patient safety metric (e.g., the goal is to have 100 percent of patients tested for the relevant genes before receiving their first dose of the drug).[6]

DISCUSSION

Protecting Against the Misuse of Information from the Genome

A topic of much discussion was preventing the misuse of genetic information and ensuring that the application of genomics in health care does not further exacerbate health disparities and discrimination. One participant asked, how can "the systemic extinction of neuroatypical persons and other marginalized groups" be prevented?

Greater legal and regulatory attention on how to prevent "the misuse of information from the genome to selectively apply our social or cultural preferences for particular groups of people or different elements of human diversity" may be essential, Baker said. As an example, the selective abortion of fetuses based on genetic screening results has essentially eliminated Down syndrome in some places around the world, he said. The Genetic Information Nondiscrimination Act was designed to help protect people from discrimination based on their genetic information. However, it does not consider how genomic information might be used to make decisions about an unborn fetus, particularly from a eugenics standpoint, he added.

An underlying issue is the flawed determination of the value of the quality of life of a member of a particular population, especially as assessed by those who are not part of that population, Baker suggested. For example, studies have found that people without disabilities rate the quality of life of people with a given disability much lower than those with the disability rate their own quality of life. It is this perception (or misperception) of the value of life that drives "what ultimately would be eugenics practices of trying to ensure that children with particular disabilities or particular elements of their identity are simply not born," he said. Cost-benefit analyses of preci-

---

[6]Thiopurines are commonly used to treat autoimmune disorders and acute lymphoblastic leukemia; however, there are various genetic interactions that can affect drug response (Fridley et al., 2010).

sion medicine interventions can take the firsthand perspectives and experiences of people living with genetic conditions into account, Baker said.

Wilkins added that current policies and practices are focused on protecting individuals, not groups of people, from misuse of genetic information. Any policy or practice solutions must start with acknowledging the country's history of eugenics and of creating structures of oppression directed at groups of people, Wilkins said, and individuals from affected groups should be engaged in developing policies and oversight mechanisms. Genetic data or presumed genetic data can be misused "to reinforce stereotypes, systems of oppression, [and] inferiority." The fears and concerns that marginalized and minoritized people have about the misuse of genetic information are valid and must not be dismissed, she said. The smaller the minority group, the greater the risk of the loss of individual data privacy, she added. Baker added that there is a belief that disparities in health are associated with "something fundamental" in the genome. A focus on the individual is the core of precision medicine. However, "a focus on the individual in terms of disparities is simply shifting the blame from the structural forces that are creating and maintaining the disparities…to the individual," emphasizing genetics and behavior and taking the focus off addressing these societal structures, he said.

The perspective that genomics is objective scientifically supports precision medicine, but Baker observed that genomics has also been "weaponized" in policies relating to individual social and cultural identity. For example, people with intersex variations and those who are transgender have been targeted, and it has become "the province of the government or a sporting body…to tell you who you are and how you fit into society, and what kinds of benefits, protections, and access are available to you," he said.

Increased efforts may be essential to educate the public and professionals about both the benefits and the limitations of genomic information, Lázaro-Muñoz said.

Capturing Racial, Ethnic, and Ancestral Identity Information

Panelists also discussed the need for new approaches for capturing data on an individual's identity. Relling said St. Jude uses the National Institutes of Health (NIH) categories for race and ethnicity and includes self-declared race and genomic ancestry data when publishing studies. Individuals who participate in the All of Us research program are asked to select which race and ethnicity categories they feel best identifies them from a list of many options, Wilkins said, which offers an alternative to the constraints of the Office of Management and Budget (OMB) categories, which NIH uses. Participants can choose as many as they want. They can also answer branching questions and select any ethnicity or nationality subgroups that correspond with how they identify. Data are compiled and still reported according to the OMB categories as required, she noted. For pharmacogenetics, focusing on the genomic variants instead of racial or ancestral identity results in clinical prescribing guidelines that are broadly applicable regardless of race or ancestry in almost all cases, Relling noted.

How the Genomics Community Can Promote Equity

As an example of the challenges of equitable use of genomic data, Relling said that the human leukocyte antigen (HLA) genotyping algorithms being used are largely based on data from individuals of European ancestry and do not provide accurate results for persons who are not of European ancestry. Although St. Jude could deliver accurate results to its patients of European ancestry, it was decided to not provide preemptive HLA genotype results to any patient at this time. The situation with HLA genotyping is a good example of how some groups currently benefit less from genomics and precision care than others, Wilkins said. Funding can help to close these types of gaps, in this case, to develop HLA genotyping algorithms in other ancestry groups so accurate results can be provided to all patients, she noted. There is a need to better integrate data on social and structural determinants of health with other health-related data, Wilkins highlighted. Precision medicine is a powerful tool for health, and the genomics community should not only develop and apply these types of tools and technologies but also participate in ensuring they reach all those who can benefit from them, Baker said.

Drawing on the St. Jude experience, Relling supported a model in which genomic testing would be embedded in institutional policies that direct best practices in care. This model reduces provider-based variability, and testing becomes routine for all patients, regardless of background, sex, race, or ancestry, she said. For example, weight, height, age, and liver and renal function are always considered when prescribing, she noted. If practice evolved such that prescribing was not done without knowledge of the patient's pharmacogenetic testing results, "then all patients would benefit from pharmacogenomics…not just the select few at academic medical centers where the physicians are trained to order pharmacogenetic tests."

5

Exploring Logistical Barriers to Genetic Testing

Highlights of Key Points Made by Individual Speakers

- Achieving full integration of genomics into primary care requires improved guidelines, clinician education, clinical decision support, EHR connectivity, transparency around costs and reimbursement, and simplification of genomic testing (e.g., one test), which could help providers more easily choose and order clinical genomic testing. (Massart)
- Genetic counselors can help primary care providers understand the nuances of genetic testing and interpretation, but improving access this way is challenging because they are not uniformly recognized as health care providers for reimbursement. (Massart)
- The processes for coding and reimbursement of genomic services have not kept up with the technological advances. Therefore, reexamination of what constitutes a genetic test may need to be considered. Restructuring the order form around the clinical problem rather than the diagnostic test could help address the issue. (Hilborne)
- Coverage decisions, coding, and reimbursement of genomic testing is complex, multidimensional, and evolving. Coverage decisions are influenced by evidence but are often driven by rules and regulations (including unspoken rules and traditions). (Quinn)

- Many payers will only reimburse guideline-endorsed tests, yet the development of practice guidelines that inform clinical decision support is not keeping pace with practitioners' needs. Professional societies could work with practitioners to develop these guidelines. (Irons, Massart)
- Patients continue to get caught up in the health care system, that was built on racism, and to address this, the health care community needs to advocate for policy change so it can improve health equity. (Henley)

In this session, speakers discussed logistical challenges to genetic testing that will need to be addressed for the full implementation of genomics in precision health care. The session was moderated by Victoria Pratt, vice president of Molecular Diagnostic Quality Assessments at Optum Genomics.

THE EFFECT OF CODING AND REIMBURSEMENT ON ACCESS

Genetic testing is complex, and the science is advancing "faster than any other area in laboratory medicine," said Lee Hilborne, senior medical director at Quest Diagnostics and professor of pathology and laboratory medicine at the David Geffen School of Medicine at the University of California, Los Angeles (UCLA). However, the processes for reporting results and reimbursing providers for services have not kept pace with the technological advances. As discussed earlier, genetic testing is a tool and obtaining a result is only the first step in the process. The tool provides value when appropriate actions can be taken based on the results. As testing technology advances and the cost of testing becomes much less of a barrier, he said, the greater challenge will be what happens after the test results become available.

System Barriers to Genetic Testing

Hilborne reviewed some of the main system barriers to access to genetic testing before discussing coding and reimbursement in depth.

Knowledge. Although there is general awareness of genetic testing, greater understanding of genetics and its role in precision medicine is needed by many providers (physicians, genetic counselors, laboratory professionals, and others), patients, payers and employers, and the public, Hilborne said.

Language. Dealing with the nomenclature of clinical laboratory testing is challenging in general, and the language of genes and genetic testing is very complicated, especially for those who do not encounter it regularly, Hilborne said. Providers and patients rely on geneticists and genetic counselors to interpret genetic testing results.

Complexity. There are multiple indications for genetic testing, including diagnostic, prognostic, or predictive testing; screening to determine carrier status; and pharmacogenetic testing for therapeutic response, Hilborne said. Genetic panels for a given condition can vary across laboratories. In addition to indication, patient history, ethnicity, known genetics, and patient preferences also come into play when choosing which test to order.

Value. The ACCE model has been used to evaluate the value of genetic tests according to *a*nalytic validity, *c*linical validity, *c*linical utility, and associated *e*thical, legal, and social implications.[1] Laboratories routinely assess analytic and clinical validity; however, establishing the clinical utility of new genetic tests has often been challenging. There may be areas in which having the ability to do genetic testing does not necessarily mean you should, Hilborne said. He added that meeting payers' criteria for clinical utility has been an impediment to coverage for some tests.

Cost. The cost of sequencing a genome has decreased significantly as the technology for sequencing has advanced, yet patient costs and reimbursement do not always reflect this. "Genetic testing remains disproportionately costly compared to other laboratory diagnostics," Hilborne said, adding that deciding whether to incur the cost of a test requires consideration of medical appropriateness (e.g., the extent to which benefit outweighs risk) and medical necessity.

Coding and Reimbursement. Early Current Procedural Terminology (CPT®) coding for molecular diagnostics required selecting a code for each of the individual laboratory procedures performed for the testing and "stacking" them. Later, gene-specific codes were created, each of which incorporated the analytical laboratory services that were previously coded separately. There are still some nonspecific codes for groups of procedures, Hilborne said, including a catchall code for molecular pathology procedures that do not have a code.

The pricing of genetic tests initially reflected that most of the testing was for individual genes and was done using the labor-intensive Sanger sequencing method. As technology advanced, multianalyte assays with algorithmic analysis became more common, and new CPT codes were created in 2015 to address the emerging multianalyte genomic sequencing procedures (GSPs). Currently, there are about 50 GSP codes, Hilborne said; however, the list is not comprehensive, and while the GSP codes identify the indication, ambiguity persists because of the range of procedures available.

---

[1] For historical information on the ACCE model see https://www.cdc.gov/genomics/gtesting/acce/index.htm (accessed December 15, 2022).

In 2017, codes were created for proprietary laboratory analyses (PLAs) that are generally specific to a particular laboratory (or manufacturer). There are currently about 350 PLA codes, and he noted that there are some payment challenges associated with these codes.

Specificity versus simplicity is on ongoing challenge for the coding of genetic testing. Complex surgical procedures (e.g., liver transplantation) generally have a single CPT code, while there are numerous codes for molecular services. Although payers and other groups have sought stream-lined solutions, he said, specificity regarding which services were performed is needed to adjudicate claims.

The reporting of genetic testing services is complex, Hilborne con-cluded. CPT is the code set recognized by the Health Insurance Portability and Accountability Act of 1996, but the coding struggles to keep pace with the evolution of the technology, he said. In addition, there are a number of ongoing efforts to provide new solutions for the challenges of cataloging and coding the ever-increasing number of genetic tests (e.g., NIH Genetic Test Registry, Palmetto MolDx DEX Registry, Concert Genetics Coding Engine).

Alluding to earlier remarks in the day, one participant asked what will happen to the ecosystem for genetic testing when a genome costs $100. Hilborne replied that the way genetic testing is considered, from the per-spective of CPT, will change as the cost shifts more toward the professional work rather than the technical work. He added that the value added by the work of genetic counselors and other genetics professionals (e.g., Ph.D. medical geneticist, physician medical geneticist) will also need to be consid-ered when discussing coding and reimbursement to ensure equitable access.

Addressing Coding and Reimbursement Challenges

Hilborne highlighted several opportunities to address these coding and reimbursement challenges and to realize the potential of genomics in preci-sion health care:

- Developing clear evidence of clinical validity and clinical utility.
- Coming to general agreement on what constitutes an appropriate genetic evaluation for a patient with a specific condition to curb fraud, waste, and abuse that emerges from uncertainty.
- Reexamining what constitutes a genetic test. Hilborne suggested that separate codes might be needed for the technical component (the sequencing) and for the analysis of the data by the laboratory professionals as well as by geneticists and others.
- Reducing the complexity of ordering genetic tests and of the results reports. Ordering could be restructured around the clinical prob-

lem rather than the genetic test (e.g., clinicians could order testing for hereditary breast and ovarian cancer rather than needing to know which specific gene tests to order). He noted that reimbursement issues regarding reflex testing would need to be addressed. For example, diagnosis codes entered to support the original test might not support downstream reflex testing.

ADDING GENOMICS TO THE PRIMARY CARE TOOLBOX

Mylynda Massart, assistant professor of family medicine at the University of Pittsburgh and founder and director of the University of Pittsburgh Medical Center (UPMC) Primary Care Precision Medicine Center, highlighted some of the many uses of genetic testing in primary care. These uses included validating the results patients receive from direct-to-consumer genetic testing; screening for hereditary cancer syndromes; pharmacogenomics for medication prescribing; prenatal carrier risk assessment; newborn screening, which is increasingly incorporating genomic sequencing; chronic disease management; polygenic risk scores; and the management of common adult genetic disorders. She shared her perspective on how to make genomics more readily accessible to primary care clinicians and others.

Barriers to the Implementation of Genomics as a Tool in Primary Care

For most individuals, primary care is the main access point in the health care system, covering urban and rural areas as well as underserved communities. There are many uses for genetic testing in primary care, Massart said, and primary care providers should be able to use genetic testing as a tool just as they use radiology as a tool (e.g., ordering and interpreting x-rays and magnetic resonance imaging without needing to consult a radiologist). If the findings indicate the need for specialized care, patients can then be referred to a specialist. She noted that medical geneticists will always be needed for expert consultation and for management of patients with rare genetic diseases or classic genetic syndromes.

There are many barriers to the implementation of genomics as a tool in primary care, Massart said. Regarding the testing itself, the availability, cost, and reimbursement of genetic testing are barriers, as is the laboratory turnaround time, which can be slow. Clinical barriers include the lack of patient access to clinical genetic testing services in general and particularly among underserved populations, the limited availability of algorithms, and a lack of randomized controlled trial data and real-world data to understand outcomes and value. There are informatics challenges, including how best to manage the huge volumes of data and how best to provide genetic testing results and point-of-care clinical decision support in the

EHR. Research-related challenges include complicated participant consent processes and an inability to integrate research and clinical care and share research information for the benefit of the patient. From an educational perspective, current and future health care professionals are not receiving training in genomics and precision medicine. Finally, she said, there are ethical, legal, and social implications of genetic testing that need to be better addressed. A question was asked about managing data security and Massart said, "The reality is that true data security is nearly impossible." The solution is to enact policies and approaches that prevent the use of an individual's genomic information against them. She added that patients should also be able to track how their data are being used and shared (e.g., for their clinical care, for research).

Addressing the Challenges in Primary Care

Massart highlighted five main areas of opportunity to enable the use of genomics as a tool in precision care:

1. **The EHR.** Orderable genetic tests need to be included in the EHR, Massart said. The EHR should also include discrete reporting of results that then triggers clinical decision support to aid in data interpretation.
2. **Cost and reimbursement.** Massart highlighted the need for transparency around the cost and reimbursement of genetic testing as well as sensible reimbursement models and clear pathways for obtaining reimbursement. Furthermore, she said, out-of-pocket costs for patients should be affordable.
3. **Guidelines and education.** Massart suggested that "genomic clinicians" are needed. These providers could integrate genomics in routine care but not necessarily be formally trained in medical genomics. She also highlighted the need for clear algorithms for use in determining who needs testing and when to test; minimal competencies for ordering genetic tests, providing pre- and posttest counseling and interpretation of test results; and increased coverage of genomics in medical education.
4. **Scalability of tools.** To provide genomics services at scale there is a need for more genetic counselors and increased diversity among genetic counselors. Other needs Massart identified included reimbursement for services provided by genetic counselors, and new models for both synchronous and asynchronous contributions from genetic counselors.
5. **Testing.** Genomic testing needs to be streamlined, Massart said, noting that the cost of sequential gene-by-gene testing is approach-

ing the cost of whole exome[2] or whole genome sequencing. She also highlighted the need for indication-driven interpretation of findings, the reporting of all actionable secondary findings to patients, and the ability to reanalyze prior sequencing data for reinterpretation as knowledge evolves.

A Stepwise Approach to Integrating Genomics into Primary Care

Achieving full integration of genomics into primary care requires improved guidelines and education, enhanced clinical decision support and EHR connectivity, better transparency of costs and reimbursement, and simplification of testing, Massart said. She outlined four models that together make up a "coordinated stepwise approach to the future" (see Figure 5-1).

Genetic Testing Utilization Clinic Model

One system-wide solution that has already proven effective in some places is genetic testing utilization clinics. These clinics, overseen by genetic counselors, work in partnership with laboratories to support clinicians and patients in accessing appropriate genetic testing. This model helps to reduce the risks of medical mistakes associated with inappropriate test selection, inadequate pre- and posttest counseling, poor utilization management, and inaccurate interpretation of test results, Massart explained. It can also help address clinicians' avoidance of ordering testing because of how overwhelming the process can be.

Hub-and-Spoke Model of Centralized Genomic Clinics Serving Primary Care

The second model, which Massart noted is currently in use at University of Pittsburgh Medical Center, establishes centralized hubs of primary care genomics expertise to serve the primary care clinics in a health system or geographic region. A strength of this model is that fewer genomic experts are needed, and she described it as a stopgap measure until the education of new primary care genomics experts can catch up with the demand. In this way, she said, there can be support for clinicians to ensure that patients get the best test, coverage, informed consent, and interpretation of results. Another strength is that each expert consultation provides opportunities to educate referring clinicians. There are weaknesses, however, including

---

[2]An exome is the sequence of all protein-coding portions, or exons, in a genome (Green, 2023).

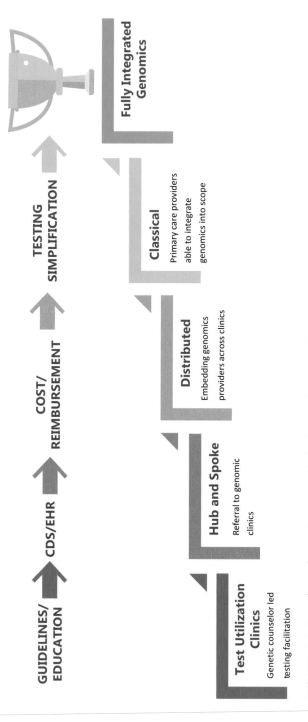

FIGURE 5-1 Coordinated stepwise approach for integrating genomics in primary care.
SOURCE: Mylynda Massart, National Academies of Sciences, Engineering, and Medicine workshop presentation, October 12, 2022.

the potential for delays in accessing services and the need to see providers who are outside the patient's medical home, which can present barriers to access, especially for underserved communities. Massart added that this model can still feel more like a specialist consultation than an embedded part of one's primary care.

Distributive Model of Embedding Genomics Providers in Primary Care

The next step would be a distributed model in which genetic counselors are embedded within primary care clinics to provide genomics expertise (similar to pharmacists, social workers, and nutritionists who work within primary care practices). Strengths of this model, Massart said, are the ability to rapidly scale, and the opportunity to relieve the primary care provider of the need to manage the nuances of genetic testing and interpretation of results. A key barrier to implementing this model, she noted, is the fact that genetic counselors are not uniformly recognized as health care providers for the purposes of reimbursement.

Integration of Genetics into the Classical Family Medicine Model

The last step discussed by Massart is the integration of genetics into the classical model of family medicine such that it becomes part of the scope of practice. Family medicine physicians are broadly trained and already manage the majority of their patients' needs, referring them to specialty care when needed. Expanding the scope of primary care and family medicine practice to include genomics will require the education of trainees and support for practicing physicians.

MEDICARE COVERAGE DECISIONS
RELATED TO GENOMIC TESTING

Bruce Quinn, an independent consultant at Bruce Quinn Associates, LLC, provided an overview of evolving national and local Medicare coverage decisions for genomic testing. One issue, he said, is that Medicare policies and rules do not always match up with Medicare data. As background he pointed out that there are no copayments for laboratory tests, including genomic tests, for those covered by Medicare, and fee schedules for laboratory tests are publicly available. Prices for new tests are initially set by the Centers for Medicare & Medicaid Services and are reset every 3 years based on a national survey of commercial insurance prices.

Data on Medicare Part B payments for laboratory testing are also made publicly available, and Quinn shared some observations based on recent data. The top 15 genomic testing codes paid by Medicare in calendar year

2020 accounted for $2.2 billion, 88 percent of genomic test payments. The most frequent test code paid by Medicare, COVID-19 polymerase chain reaction (PCR) testing, accounted for nearly $1 billion of that total. Of the remaining $1.5 billion paid for the other 14 codes, 42 percent was attributable to proprietary single tests (e.g., Cologuard®, Oncotype DX®). Another 32 percent of the remaining $1.5 billion was paid out for what Quinn said are "heavily abused codes." He described how he used publicly available information from the Department of Justice (e.g., code patterns used by laboratories that were indicted) and Medicare laboratory claims data for his analysis. These laboratories often have nondescript names (e.g., ABC Lab, Best Lab) and primarily bill Tier 2 CPT codes (especially 81408 and 81407 for sequence analysis of genes associated with very rare disorders), and code 87798 (a nonspecific code for detection of pathogens by PCR), Quinn said. He noted that the six codes most frequently used by these laboratories for fraudulent Medicare billing are used infrequently by well-known laboratories. If payments for codes that are "heavily abused" are excluded, proprietary tests now comprise 60 percent of non-COVID-19-testing Medicare payments, indicating that they have done very well in the current Medicare system, he said.

National and Local Coverage Decisions for Genomics Tests

National Coverage Decisions

Quinn discussed three main Medicare national coverage decisions for genomics tests. In 2014, CMS issued a decision to cover Cologuard®, a DNA-based screening test for colon cancer that is done on a self-collected and submitted fecal sample. The price for Cologuard® is about $500, and the product is advertised heavily to the public. Currently, he said, it is one of the highest paid codes in Medicare (about $300 million).

In 2018, CMS issued a decision for next-generation sequencing in cancer. This decision guarantees national coverage for next-generation sequencing-based companion diagnostics for cancer if they are U.S. Food and Drug Administration (FDA) approved, Quinn said, adding that the intent is to incentivize developers to seek FDA approval. Currently, the decision blocks the use of the same test more than once, which presents a barrier to the use of liquid biopsy tests to detect minimal residual disease or recurrence.

In 2021, CMS issued a national coverage decision for liquid biopsy for colorectal cancer screening. Per the decision, CMS will cover any FDA-approved blood-based colorectal cancer screening test that achieves 74 percent sensitivity and 90 percent specificity. At the time of the workshop, no test meeting this standard had been approved by FDA. Quinn pointed out how this decision again uses policy to incentivize development and approval of a test with important public health implications.

Local Coverage Decisions

There are three Medicare Administrative Contractors (MACs) who issue local coverage decisions for genomic tests for their designated geographic areas, and they behave in different ways, Quinn said.

The National Government Services (NGS) MAC system covers Minnesota, Wisconsin, Illinois, New York, and the states of New England. Quinn said NGS MAC has strict policies and makes far fewer genomic test payments than other MACs (per capita or per million Medicare beneficiaries). As a result, fraudulent laboratories tend to avoid these states and NGS MAC has essentially "zero fraudulent payments."

The Novitas system covers Texas and the surrounding states, as well as Pennsylvania and Florida. After being "battered by high abnormal payments," which Quinn said likely reached $1 billion, Novitas is drafting very strict new local coverage decisions. For example, they will not cover any cardiology gene testing, and will only cover gene tests for cancer that are endorsed by guidelines.

The MolDx system covers the rest of the country and was established to make local coverage decisions specifically for molecular diagnostic tests. Quinn described MolDx as a "complex body of policies, rules, tech assessments, websites, [and] databases." He noted that MolDx has comparatively liberal policies for the coverage of minimal residual disease testing, pharmacogenetics, and hereditary testing. For pharmacogenetics, for example, MolDx covers all testing recommended by CPIC guidelines.

Reform and Regulation

The Medicare Coverage for Innovative Technology (MCIT) program, proposed by the Trump administration in 2020, called for Medicare to cover any device, including tests, designated by FDA as a breakthrough device, Quinn said. Coverage would be automatic and would initially be for 4 years. MCIT was repealed by the Biden administration in 2021, in favor of a new program called Transitional Coverage for Emerging Technology. Quinn noted there have been several town hall meetings and reports, but no proposal has been released (Fleisher and Blum, 2022; Zeitler et al., 2022).

Coverage decisions, coding, and reimbursement are "very complex and multidimensional," Quinn concluded. They are influenced by evidence but exist primarily in a policy world driven by rules and regulations, as well as unspoken rules and traditions.

DISCUSSION

Developing Guidelines to Support
Clinical Decision Making and Coverage of Testing

Irons and Massart discussed that the practice guidelines that inform clinical decision support are generally written by professional societies, and that the writing of guidelines for presymptomatic patients is not keeping pace with practitioners' needs. Many payers will only reimburse guideline-endorsed tests, Irons said, suggesting that professional societies should work with practitioners to develop guidelines. Family medicine and primary care doctors should be involved in generating guidelines, Massart said, adding that her clinic is currently developing a guideline for the evaluation and management of connective tissue disorders in the primary care setting, including identifying patients for genetic testing. The lack of reimbursement by Medicare and commercial insurance companies is a barrier for patient access to emerging precision medicine applications, Massart said. Even patients with insurance will incur out-of-pocket costs if services are not covered, she added, creating a situation where "only those with means get access." An additional challenge is that guidelines on competencies in genetics and genomics that have been long endorsed by the American Academy of Family Physicians are not being integrated into family medicine training, Massart said.

Closing the Policy and Knowledge Gaps that Affect Equitable Access

Much of the discussion focused on addressing the issues that affect equitable access to genetic testing. One participant noted that "policy always lags far behind the evidence" and that this gap mostly affects those who are already underserved by the health system. Because the United States does not have a national health care system, Massart said, addressing this gap will require "a multipronged commitment across the country to solve these challenges and a [prioritization of] policy, protection, access, and equity." She said that lack of coverage for services is a barrier to access, and many patients will not benefit from precision medicine services until those services have uniform coverage by payers. Further, when only those with means can access new services, the data collected are not representative of the larger population and these data often inform implementation, algorithm development, and coverage decisions.

One participant raised the issue of coverage under Medicaid and access to genetic services for those who receive their health care at safety net clinics, pointing out that women now have better access to cancer germline testing at safety net clinics, but they still face challenges getting genetic counseling and follow-up care if they test positive. Hilborne said that Medicaid programs vary by state, and it is important to start having discussions about what policies and processes need to change to ensure access under Medicaid.

Feero said that rurality also presents access challenges that lead to disparities. "In rural states that are less well off, budgets are extremely tight [and] chronic disease is extremely prevalent," and he said that genetics and genomics become low priority. In these areas the gap in access to new technologies continues to widen. Massart praised the work of those in the National Health Service Corps and others serving patients in the nation's Federally Qualified Health Centers and suggested that advances in telemedicine can be used to help close gaps in access to care *if* rural areas can get equitable access to the necessary digital technology and services.

There are knowledge gaps among providers, Hilborne said, especially regarding new technologies and approaches. Patients can receive care that is technically appropriate, but opportunities for accessing more advanced care can be missed. It is essential to find ways to get information to providers and patients, especially in underserved communities, so they can make informed decisions about their care.

Advocating for Action on Systemic Change

Henley emphasized that the care those in underserved communities receive is not only a result of the level of knowledge or skill of providers. "Our health care system was built on racism," she said, and racism and disparities in health care persist today. The health care system has been mired in bureaucratic "red tape" for decades and decades, which has sowed divisiveness. As a result, patients get "caught up in the system," Henley said, and she described it as "tragic" and "embarrassing" that people of color are still treated differently when seeking care in the United States. This will continue, she said, until more individuals in the medical community say enough is enough.

"Everyone, in every position, needs to advocate for change," Henley said. She urged participants to use their voices to advocate for action by those who are in positions to make change. This includes policy makers, members of Congress, and those responsible for creating the red tape. Valuable time is being wasted in meeting after meeting, year after year, as the same issues are discussed and nothing changes. Instead, she said, it is time to change the conversation and focus on "changing the health care system and pushing our policy makers to do better."

6

System-Level Challenges and Opportunities

Highlights of Key Points Made by Individual Speakers

- Partnering with community and faith leaders can promote trust in science and medicine by providing sustained outreach to underserved minority communities. Deploying culturally congruent "honest brokers" to be trusted sources of information about the health benefits of genomics can help address community concerns about participating in research. (Cunningham)
- Payment models that incentivize high-quality care and patient outcomes instead of rewarding volume and productivity are needed, as primary care providers have little to no time for integrating genomics into the patient encounter. (Zazove)
- Structured genomic data and clinical decision support tools that are integrated with the EHR are needed to enable genomics as part of routine care. (Kaul, Zazove)
- Medical school and residency curricula need to keep pace with advances in genomics so future providers can be sufficiently trained in these areas. (Kaul)
- Areas to improve that may lead to better reimbursement for laboratories include reimbursement rates for genetic testing, approval of payment for tests that are considered experimental, reimbursement for tests beyond those recommended by clinical practice guidelines, and reimbursement for interpretation of sequencing results. (Kaul)

- Given clinical care time constraints and varying levels of clinical experience with genetic risk, it may make more sense to build systems that fit and support the provider's expertise rather than the other way around. (Maxwell)
- ACMG ACTion (ACT) Sheets, which provide immediate actionable information to the clinician, could be a model adapted to cover incidental findings that patients receive from direct-to-consumer products or other genetic tests. (Irons)

The final panel session, moderated by Greg Feero, professor in the Department of Community and Family Medicine at Geisel School of Medicine and faculty at Maine Dartmouth Family Medicine Residency Program, examined system-level barriers to the widespread adoption of genomics in health care. Topics discussed spanned raising patient awareness of genomics, getting patients tested, laboratory concerns, delivery of results, and medical management based on the results.

PROMOTING PATIENT ENGAGEMENT IN GENOMICS

Tshaka Cunningham, chief science officer and cofounder of Polaris Genomics and executive director of the Faith-Based Genetic Research Institute (FBGRI), discussed how FBGRI is working to empower minority communities with the knowledge needed to engage in and benefit from genomics and precision medicine.

For many in minority communities, trust in medical research is lacking because of a long history of discrimination and exploitation, Cunningham said. One well-known example of this is the U.S. Public Health Service Syphilis Study at Tuskegee that ran from 1932 to 1972 and had detrimental health effects on African Americans in rural Alabama.[1] Another example is Henrietta Lacks' tumor cells, taken without her knowledge or consent to establish the HeLa cell line,[2] that has been used in the research and development of numerous medical products that have earned the pharmaceutical industry billions of dollars, with no acknowledgment or compensation to her family. In addition, African American patients have experienced, and continue to experience, "countless instances of health disparities."

To promote trust in science and medicine, FBGRI is partnering with community and faith leaders to provide sustained outreach to underserved minority communities through ongoing in-person events at local churches

---

[1] See https://www.cdc.gov/tuskegee/index.html (accessed January 9, 2023).
[2] See https://www.britannica.com/biography/Henrietta-Lacks (accessed January 9, 2023).

and other community-serving institutions, as well as online resources. He pointed out that, for many African Americans, the church has long been considered a safe space where they can receive information from their pastors, community leaders, and other trusted individuals. FBGRI deploys "honest broker communicators," including people of color from the communities and scientists of color to discuss the health benefits of genomics and precision medicine and to address concerns about participating in research (e.g., fears about how a patient's data might be shared or used against them). "People really respond to people who are from their community; there's an instant trust bond there," he said. When people have a better understanding, there is greater engagement and participation. Another strategy for building trust in communities could be ensuring that the genomics infrastructure and industry support innovators who are people of color in developing new technologies and products. This, Cunningham said, could fill a current gap and could help individuals in these communities see themselves in all aspects of genomics.

In summary, Cunningham listed three opportunities for promoting trust and engaging communities in genomics:

- Highlight the health benefits that minority patients have seen thus far that are attributable to advances in science and biomedical research.
- Provide culturally congruent "honest brokers" that can be a trusted source of scientific information for African Americans and other minorities.
- Address racism at the highest levels in academia, industry, and government to create a truly level playing field for scientists of color in the United States.

GENOMICS IN FAMILY MEDICINE PRACTICE

Philip Zazove, professor emeritus and past chair of the Department of Family Medicine at the University of Michigan, shared his perspective as a family medicine physician on the main systems issues that are affecting the uptake of genomics in primary care and offered some potential solutions.

Quality of Care

Primary care providers have, on average, 15 to 30 minutes to spend with each patient to address the reasons for their visit, Zazove said. He noted that just covering the relevant preventive services recommended by the U.S. Preventive Services Task Force takes far longer than that. Additional time is needed for patients with multiple conditions and for patients whose health is affected by social factors that need to be addressed. When it comes to integrating genomics into the encounter, "there is no time."

To address this, Zazove said that new paradigms of care are needed that shift the focus toward population health and that emphasize the quality of care each patient receives rather than the number of patients each provider sees in an hour. He suggested that this shift in practice could result in having more time available to incorporate genomics.

Institutional and System Factors

Zazove reiterated that when institutions and systems emphasize volume (e.g., seeing as many patients as possible) and productivity (e.g., money generated) there is little incentive for spending time addressing issues such as genomics. Another barrier is that genomic data are not widely integrated into EHR systems. There are no pop-up notifications to alert the physician that the patient is at risk for a genetic disorder or to recommend appropriate genetic tests. Zazove said it can also be very difficult for the primary care providers to get information about the patient's genetic history and test results. He noted that genetics clinics have staff dedicated to gathering and reviewing each patient's genetic history and test results, and family medicine practices generally do not have the resources to do this.

One solution, Zazove said, is to incorporate identification of at-risk patients and recommendations for genetic testing into the EHR. Another is to implement tools such as the Inherited Risk Evaluation Tool (InheRET),[3] developed at the University of Michigan, which facilitates risk assessment and identification of patients who should be tested. He also highlighted the need to provide financial incentives for health systems to implement the infrastructure needed to support genomics in primary care.

Scope of Primary Care

Zazove said most of what family medicine providers see in their practices are multifactorial conditions for which there are not yet genomic explanations or actions to be taken (e.g., diabetes, congestive heart failure, depression, hypertension). Practices also deal with the health effect of patients' socioeconomic and environmental conditions and the effects of having multiple diseases. On average, only about five patients out of a typical panel of 2,000, for example, would have genomic findings associated with *BRCA* or Lynch syndrome. "There is no real solution here," Zazove said, other than to "recognize that what we see in family medicine and primary care is very different than what the specialists see." What might

---

[3]See https://www.inheret.com/Pages/Home# (accessed December 14, 2022).

work for specialist practices does not necessarily work for primary care practices, he said.

Complexity of Primary Care

"Primary care is incredibly complex [and] not well understood by most," Zazove said. The breadth of services that primary care practitioners provide every day makes it very difficult to stay current on the many advances in the field of genomics.

Again, a solution here is to add functionality to the EHR to automatically identify at-risk patients and provide guidance on testing, he said. He also noted that residents receive training in genomics and often have more up-to-date knowledge than many faculty, and he suggested using resources such as the Society of Teachers of Family Medicine to ensure that providers stay up to date.

ISSUES FOR THE LABORATORY

Karen Kaul, chair of the Department of Pathology and Laboratory Medicine at NorthShore University HealthSystem and clinical professor of pathology at the University of Chicago Pritzker School of Medicine, said DNA- and RNA-based testing have "revolutionized" the practice of medicine. For example, somatic genomic testing of cancer cells aids diagnosis and informs treatment decisions, and germline testing has many applications, including diagnosis of genetic disorders, assessment of risk of heritable cancers, and pharmacogenomics. Molecular diagnostics have transformed microbiology, and she mentioned COVID-19 molecular diagnostics as an example. Although progress in genomics has advanced patient care, there are systemic barriers to the uptake of genomics, and Kaul discussed these challenges and potential solutions from a laboratory perspective.

Education of Clinical Providers

A challenge for the medical education system is that the field of genomics is advancing very rapidly. Medical school and residency curricula are not keeping pace, and future providers are not being sufficiently trained in these areas. Kaul offered several solutions, which she said should be implemented broadly and equitably. These included ongoing training for practicing providers, training champions in primary care (e.g., a hub-and-spoke model of expertise) and developing EHR-embedded tools that enable providers to incorporate genomic testing into routine care.

EHR Functionality

As discussed by previous speakers, genomics is complex, and greater functionality in the EHR could help overcome some of the practice barriers and support research. EHRs need to contain structured genomic data, Kaul said, and should facilitate the identification of family groupings and connections. Ordering genomic tests is also complex, and EHRs should enable ordering of the appropriate test and any necessary reflex testing and facilitate any required consent and preauthorization. The display and accessibility of genetic testing results present barriers as results are generally scanned into a PDF file that is uploaded to the EHR. Results need to be "intelligible, actionable, and ideally, make them live," she said. For example, NorthShore University HealthSystem has built a just-in-time pop-up function into its EHR that alerts providers ordering a drug if there are relevant pharmacogenomics data available. The EHR should also alert providers to the existence of results for germline testing to eliminate unnecessary reordering of these "once-in-a-lifetime" tests. EHR vendors are working to incorporate these types of tools, she said, but needed functionality is still generally lacking.

Reimbursement of Testing

One systemic testing-related barrier that has been discussed, Kaul reiterated, is the need for reimbursement of the time spent by genetic counselors, primary care providers, or other practitioners to explain the testing and results to patients. Laboratories also face reimbursement challenges as reimbursement rates for genetic testing are often low. Tests are frequently considered to be experimental, and reimbursement is denied. Some payers only reimburse tests that are recommended by clinical practice guidelines, but these guidelines often lag behind practice. Kaul also noted that, although CPT codes have been added to the clinical laboratory fee schedule, there is no reimbursement for the interpretation of the sequencing results by laboratory professionals.

Regulatory Issues

There are also regulatory concerns for laboratories that conduct genomic tests. The number of FDA-approved molecular diagnostics for microbiology is increasing, Kaul said, which she said helps to combat the type of fraud discussed by Quinn. However, most genetics and cancer testing are still done using tests developed by each individual laboratory. Clinical laboratories, and laboratory-developed tests (LDTs), are regulated by CMS under the Clinical Laboratory Improvement Amendments (CLIA)

Act. The level of FDA oversight of LDTs has long been debated, Kaul said. Most recently, the Verifying Accurate Leading-Edge IVCT Development Act of 2022 would require that all laboratory testing be reviewed by FDA, which Kaul said could increase the cost of LDTs (which she noted are already expensive) and reduce patient access. She explained that FDA regulates laboratory test kits, while CLIA assesses the quality of the entire laboratory testing process (which might include a kit) and having FDA review LDTs would be redundant with CLIA. Discussions are ongoing, and she said that regulatory issues need to be considered as genomic testing becomes more widely implemented in routine patient care.

THE COMPLEX IMPLICATIONS OF GENETIC TESTING

Kara Maxwell, assistant professor of medicine at the Perelman School of Medicine of the University of Pennsylvania, discussed several broad system-level barriers to the uptake of genomics using cancer genetics as a case example. Management of patients with identified genetic risks has become increasingly complex and, she said, "There is not a one-size-fits-all approach."

Patient Genetic Knowledge and Testing Venues

Patients can receive genetic test results that indicate an increased risk for cancer in a variety of care delivery settings, Maxwell said, and it is important to recognize that the level of knowledge the patient comes away with varies with the setting.

In a traditional genetic testing setting for cancer risk, patients receive pretest counseling, relevant tests are ordered, and results are explained in posttest counseling. This is facilitated by a genetic counselor, and possibly a cancer genetics physician, which Maxwell noted are providers that have the most knowledge to impart in this area. A patient might also be tested at the point of care. For example, the patient's oncologist orders the test and delivers the results, possibly with the assistance of a genetic counselor. Findings of a mutation associated with increased risk of cancer can also be found incidentally, such as germline mutations identified during reproductive planning in association with a prenatal geneticist. Tumor testing ordered by an oncologist and intended to inform treatment decisions can also turn up incidental findings. Incidental findings of increased cancer risk are also returned to participants in research studies, with no particular provider associated to impart information about the findings. Finally, direct-to-consumer genetic testing presents new challenges for imparting knowledge as it provides results directly to the individual who was tested.

Medical Management of Genetic Testing Results Is Complex

Genetic testing for cancer risk is not simply about assessing if a patient is at increased risk; it is also about what can be done to mitigate that risk, Maxwell said. Medical management of cancer risk associated with a genetic mutation varies in complexity over the life span and is relative to the patient's overall health status. For example, Maxwell said that a woman who is a *BRCA* mutation carrier, but who is otherwise healthy, might continue to have breast cancer screenings across her lifetime but would also be considered for surgical interventions such as risk-reducing salpingo-oophorectomy between ages 35 and 45. Preimplantation genetic diagnosis would be relevant for persons of childbearing potential with known genetic cancer risks. Pancreatic cancer screening would be most relevant for those over age 55 who are at increased risk for hereditary pancreatic cancer. Urgent decisions regarding possible cancer treatment must be made at all ages. Discussions of addressing barriers should consider not just barriers to testing, but to providing appropriate care following testing.

Genomics Expertise Varies Among Clinical Providers

Patients can receive care for their genetic concerns from a range of providers with varying levels of genetic expertise. Expertise stems not only from training but from clinical experience. For example, Maxwell said that a genetic counselor is trained in genetic risk and counseling, and between 5 and 50 percent of their patients will have a genetic mutation (depending on the context of their practice). An oncologist is trained in the clinical management of cancer, and depending on the tumor type, between 1 and 20 percent or more of their patients will have a genetic mutation. Primary care physicians are trained in clinical management focused on risk reduction. They see patients with a wide range of conditions, and generally less than 1 percent of the patients they see will have a genetic mutation (can be higher depending on the ethnicity of the practice population). It is not realistic to expect that a primary care provider would have the same level of expertise as a genetic counselor because they do not see as many patients with genetic mutations in their practice. "We need to rely on the levels of expertise that people have, and make systems fit their expertise, not the other way around," Maxwell said.

DISCUSSION

Telemedicine

Panelists discussed using telemedicine to facilitate access to genetic services. One challenge for telemedicine is the need for genetic counselors to be licensed in the state where the patient is. While not easy, Maxwell said, it is possible for genetic counselors to be licensed in all states. She noted that all counselors in the telegenetics program at the University of Pennsylvania are licensed in all 50 states. Telehealth has enabled many people to get care they could not have received otherwise, Zazove said. He noted that his primary care practice in Michigan is 35 minutes from the Ohio border and many of their patients come from Ohio; however, the practice cannot conduct telehealth visits with patients in Ohio, which presents a problem.

Another challenge noted was that patients often need in-person physical evaluations. Maxwell said this is an infrequent barrier as many conditions do not require a physical exam. She emphasized that the occasional need for a physical exam should not stop the deployment of telegenetics care, especially to rural areas. Zazove agreed, and said only 5 to 10 percent of the physical exams they conduct reveal an abnormal finding. Further, once a patient has had an exam, and testing has been ordered, follow-up counseling can be done via telemedicine. Kaul and Cunningham reiterated the importance of telemedicine for genetic counseling, highlighting concerns about the shortage of genetic counselors. Telemedicine can be used for both pretest counseling and posttest review of results, Kaul said, though the training pipeline of genetic counselors will need attention.

Direct-to-Consumer Genetic Testing

Direct-to-consumer genetic testing is extremely popular, Irons said, and people are presenting at their primary care practice with concerning results in hand (e.g., a cancer gene mutation) wanting to know what to do. Or alternatively, they receive results that could instigate preventative action, but they do not tell their provider and later need treatment for an advanced-stage disease.

Maxwell expressed her concern that people (including some physicians) do not understand direct-to-consumer genetic testing, and misinformation abounds. Test panels vary, and people often do not understand which genetic variants are included in the test they took, and which are not, or that the lack of a finding ("being negative") does not mean lack of risk. Maxwell shared her concern that regulation of direct-to-consumer genetic tests is limited.[4] As a provider, "If you haven't seen a report, you have no idea what your patient has been tested for," she said.

Zazove said he commonly sees patients who are worried because they took a genetic test and they "have the gene." In the vast majority of cases, the findings are not significant, but they cause a lot of anxiety. He suggested there could be a clearinghouse where people could easily get free information about their test results. Cunningham described similar personal experiences, and said better education about genetic testing is needed. He mentioned that the UK National Health Service (NHS) has a genomics educational program for providers.[5] He also reiterated the need for more genetic counselors and the increased use of telemedicine for counseling.

Irons recalled a prior roundtable workshop on direct-to-consumer testing[6] and relayed a story shared by an individual who found out she was a *BRCA1* mutation carrier on a Friday afternoon and "spent the weekend with Dr. Google" because she could not get in touch with her doctor. By Monday she was extremely anxious, but her physician referred her to a genetic counselor who was able to give her information about her results. Engaging Google and health systems could be one strategy for ensuring that helpful information about genetic testing—and what to do when you get your results—is available to people searching for it online, Irons suggested.

Maxwell said that the University of Pennsylvania does have information posted online, as do other research institutions. Unfortunately, she added, it is not possible to ensure that the people searching get to the most reliable websites. Kaul cautioned that providing more information on the Internet also does not eliminate the risk that a person will assume they are not at risk because they are "negative." A participant suggested that direct-to-consumer testing is "an opportunity for people to enter into genetics," and presents an opportunity not only for patient education and engagement but also for provider education as well. Feero stated, "In many ways [consumer genomics] forced conversations about accuracy, clinical validity, [and] clinical utility that needed to happen," as well as the regulation of genetic testing and how data moves around in the system.

---

[4]For more information on FDA oversight of direct-to-consumer genetic testing see https://www.fda.gov/medical-devices/in-vitro-diagnostics/direct-consumer-tests (accessed January 4, 2023).

[5]For more information on the Health Education England Genomics Education Programme see https://www.genomicseducation.hee.nhs.uk/ (accessed January 4, 2023).

[6]See https://nap.nationalacademies.org/catalog/25713/exploring-the-current-landscape-of-consumer-genomics-proceedings-of-a (accessed December 14, 2022).

Secondary Uses of Genetic Data

Concerns about secondary uses of individuals' genetic data for research or commercial product development were discussed. In his moderator role, Feero pointed out that the Geisinger Health System entered into a research partnership with Regeneron that he said was novel and very transparent. He noted that secondary uses are often not as transparent.

Cunningham emphasized the need for diversity in clinical studies and in biobanking of samples for future uses. A look back at the history of genetic research shows that much of it was not conducted with diversity goals in mind, he said, and the clinical studies done were often not representative of the population. As a result, variants of significance for different populations, especially minority populations, are not known, and many of the genetic tests on the market are therefore not broadly applicable. The NIH All of Us program emphasizes diversity in its data collection, as does the UK Biobank, and he called upon the pharmaceutical research community to commit resources to building a more inclusive data set. Maxwell highlighted the foresight of the Department of Veterans Affairs (VA) health care system in establishing a diverse DNA biobank in 2010, the Million Veteran Program. Thus far, this program has done single nucleotide polymorphism genotyping and whole exome sequencing for over 800,000 veterans, and within the program, 25 percent of participants are self-identified racial minorities, she said. Cunningham agreed, adding that VA was very intentional in designing an outreach and recruitment strategy for minority veterans. He added that the lesson learned here is "If you really put in the time and effort, you can see the results."

Identifying Models of Success at the Systems Level

In addition to the VA's Million Veteran Program, panelists discussed whether there are other examples of successful integration of genomics into clinical care at the systems level that could be shared. Zazove suggested the InheRET program is one such example, which was discussed above. Zazove and Cunningham said they were unaware of other examples at the health systems level, although there likely were some. Maxwell mentioned the Flatiron[7] model of engaging multiple health care systems in integrating their oncology data for real-world clinical trials. She noted that there are institutional review board challenges to be addressed when combining data across health care systems. There are also barriers to sharing data across health care systems, and she again raised the issue of genetic and genomic

---

[7]Flatiron is a company that aims to learn from the experiences of individuals with cancer. See https://flatiron.com/about-us/ (accessed February 6, 2023).

data being stored in Portable Document Format (PDF) form. She suggested that natural language processing and artificial intelligence technologies could be used to extract data in PDFs and integrate it directly into the EHR in a format that could facilitate sharing across systems.

Opportunities for Incorporating Genomics in Clinical Care

Panelists and members of the roundtable suggested a variety of actions that could help promote the adoption of genomics in health care and precision medicine.

- **Enabling multistate telemedicine licensing.** Maxwell said state lines should not be barriers for telegenetics and suggested developing a road map to guide practices through the process of obtaining licensure across multiple states.
- **Increasing genetic and genomic literacy.** Cunningham highlighted the need for "genomics education for all," emphasizing that educational initiatives should be equitably implemented. He suggested that the National Academies could have a role in this, and that federal agencies should support educational initiatives. One approach, for example, is the training of community ambassadors to serve as honest broker communicators about genomics.
- **Supporting physicians in implementing genomics in practice.** Zazove said that health systems need to support the implementation of genomics in clinical care by increasing genomic functionality in the EHR and by adopting models of care that allow physicians to spend the time needed to equitably incorporate genomics into patient care and help patients get the services they need. This could also enable systems to reach out to undeserved communities who typically do not benefit from genomics advances.
- **Partnering with patients and families.** A participant said health systems should engage patients in an advisory capacity on the development of genomics programs and population sequencing efforts. She emphasized the value of patients sharing their stories, and the importance of developing "a true reciprocal relationship" that provides value back to patients and communities. Cunningham agreed that community participation is extremely valuable, but he noted again the need to build trust as concerns persist about how data could be misused. It is important to provide tangible benefits back to the community, and there can be a role for compensation. He mentioned public benefit corporations as a potential model, explaining that participants are awarded shares for their data contributions and can profit financially if their data are ever sold. Goto

said that family organizations are valuable resources that should be engaged. She described how she worked with the Alaska state affiliate of the national Family Voices organization to develop a curriculum to train navigators in rare care. Partnerships with these organizations could help to disseminate information about genetics and genomics to families in communities. She also noted the need to understand the everyday issues families face, such as helping aging parents navigate the health system and the growing population of children who are cared for by grandparents. Even the routine task of using a kiosk to check in for laboratory testing can be challenging.

- **Expanding the availability of information on rapid actions to take when patients receive testing results.** Irons pointed out that the American College of Medical Genetics and Genomics (ACMG) developed ACTion (ACT) Sheets decades ago to advise clinicians on immediate actions to take when a genetic condition is identified through newborn screening.[8] ACT Sheets are also now available for genomic findings from other types of genetic testing. She suggested that this type of model could be adapted to cover incidental findings patients receive from direct-to-consumer products or other genetic tests. These could be useful to both the patient and their physician. Martin said ACMG has issued ACT Sheets for some secondary findings and has worked in partnership with the ClinGen actionability groups. She said that synergy between these groups is important as it minimizes duplication of efforts. Maxwell agreed and said that the experts who serve on the individual ClinGen panels are passionate about their disease area and would likely be willing to help and could easily map out the rapid actions to be taken when someone receives a genetic testing result.

---

[8] For more information on ACMG ACT Sheets see https://www.acmg.net/ACMG/Medical-Genetics-Practice-Resources/ACT_Sheets_and_Algorithms.aspx (accessed January 4, 2023).

7

The Future of Genomics in Precision Health Care

The final session of the workshop considered what genomics in health care will look like in the coming decades and how the field might get there (summarized in Box 7-1) and concluded with reflections on the highlights of each session presented by Christa Martin, chief scientific officer, Geisinger, and professor and director, Autism & Developmental Medical Institute (summarized in Box 7-2).

ACHIEVING WIDESPREAD ADOPTION OF GENOMICS IN CLINICAL CARE

David Ledbetter, professor, University of Florida College of Medicine-Jacksonville, and former chief scientific officer at Geisinger, highlighted possible actions to help achieve the vision of embedding genomics into clinical practice to advance the delivery of precision care.

Removing Key Obstacles

The Cost of Genome Sequencing

In the future, the cost of genome sequencing and analysis will become more affordable and have faster turnaround times for clinicians, Ledbetter said. Although talk of "the $100 to $200 genome" can dominate conversations, Ledbetter reminded participants the $200 genome announced by Illumina is essentially the list price of the reagents used. As discussed by Ashley (Chapter 2), the cost of sequencing a genome has decreased signifi-

BOX 7-1
Perspectives on the Future of Genomics

Observations:
- The United States lags on the implementation of genomics in clinical care. (Ledbetter)
- Some genomes that are sequenced for a specific purpose (e.g., trio genome sequencing for pediatric neurodevelopmental disorders) are not being saved or further interpreted for the benefit of the individual's overall health (that is, they are "lost"). (Ledbetter)

Predictions for the future of genomics:
- Costs of genome sequencing will become affordable, and faster turn-around times will make the use of genomic results in clinical care practical. (Ledbetter)
- Genome sequencing will generally be done once in an individual's life-time and reanalyzed repeatedly, as clinical needs warrant and perhaps routinely as part of an annual physical. (Ledbetter)
- There will be a range of opportunities across the life span for individuals to have their genome sequenced (e.g., preconception screening, prenatal testing, newborn screening, germline sequencing concurrent with tumor sequencing). (Ledbetter)

Some health systems are taking the lead in translating genomics into practice by
- Making deep tumor sequencing widely available and supporting clinicians in using the data provided (Compton-Phillips),
- Integrating genomic tools at the point of care to identify individuals who would benefit from genetic testing (Compton-Phillips),
- Conducting studies of providing liquid biopsy in the primary care setting (Compton-Phillips),
- Embedding pharmacogenomics information into the EHR and developing decision support tools for clinicians (Compton-Phillips),
- Taking an implementation science approach to whole genome sequencing (i.e., learning by doing) (Compton-Phillips), and
- Developing the computing infrastructure to support the storage, sharing, and reanalysis of the vast volumes of sequencing data that will be generated. (Compton-Phillips)

This list is the rapporteurs' summary of points made by the individual speakers identified, and the statements have not been endorsed or verified by the National Academies of Sciences, Engineering, and Medicine. They are not intended to reflect a consensus among workshop participants.

cantly, but there are significant capital equipment costs and separate costs associated with analysis of the results that cannot be forgotten. A clinical diagnostic whole genome test still costs several thousand dollars today, Ledbetter said. Costs can be reduced with volume and batching, and he predicted that a whole genome sequence could be in the range of $500 in the coming years. A question for consideration, he said, is, "How cheap does it have to get?" He suggested comparing the value of a whole genome sequence, which would likely be done once in a person's lifetime, to that of other medical testing such as magnetic resonance imaging.

Sequenced Once, Analyzed Repeatedly

Today, knowing which genetic test to order for a patient can be very complicated, and physicians often order a single gene test and/or a gene panel. "Genome sequencing will become the universal genetic test," Ledbetter predicted. He suggested that, in the next 5 to 10 years, an individual's genome will be sequenced once, via a single test with a single CPT code, and then it will be reanalyzed as needed. Whole genome sequencing can also overcome some of the shortcomings of other methods in detecting repeat expansion disorders, such as fragile X syndrome (Ibañez et al., 2022).

In addition, turnaround times for whole genome sequencing and analysis will be 24 to 72 hours, Ledbetter predicted. Historically, the lack of urgency by genetics professionals in returning genetic test results has been counterproductive, negatively affecting their clinical usefulness and clinicians' perceptions of their value. For example, in the 1980s it took 6 weeks to receive the results of amniocentesis chromosome analysis, which Ledbetter described as an unnecessary delay. The work of Kingsmore and colleagues in returning whole genome sequencing results to the NICU in 50 hours has demonstrated the potential utility of whole genome sequencing for clinical care (Saunders et al., 2012).

Multiple Opportunities for Genome Sequencing

Genome sequencing will be done at various points across the life span, Ledbetter said. For example, whole genome sequencing can be done for preconception screening in place of expanded carrier screening of parents, and for prenatal screening, using cell-free DNA or fetal cells, he said. As one example, he noted a health system in Israel that is considering offering free whole genome sequencing to couples in a preconception setting as an incentive for delivering at their hospital instead of their competitors' hospital. As another example, Ledbetter said that for many patients with cancer, it is now recommended that germline sequencing be done concurrently with tumor sequencing, and the sequences compared to aid with interpretation.

There are a variety of pilot programs launching to study the use of whole genome sequencing for newborn screening. Ledbetter mentioned the GUARDIAN program in the United States,[1] which is planning to enroll 100,000 newborns, and another program to be launched in 2023 by Genomics England that he said plans to sequence genomes for 100,000 newborns per year. As discussed above, the ability to rapidly return whole genome sequencing results for patients in the NICU has been demonstrated. Ledbetter said that whole genome sequencing for all undiagnosed disease patients in the NICU and pediatric intensive care unit could save lives and reduce the length of the patient's hospital stay. In addition, Ledbetter said that some payers, including Geisinger, are now covering trio exome sequencing[2] as a more efficient alternative to chromosome microarray for patients with autism spectrum disorder and other pediatric neurodevelopmental disorders.

A question for the future is how often the interpretation of one's genome should be updated (e.g., reinterpret variants, check against updates to the ClinVar database). Ledbetter suggested that a person's annual physical exam could coincide with an annual genome checkup. An additional challenge for the future may be equity of access to genomic advances. One participant suggested that organic implementation could lead to more inequity in the health system because only those individuals who live near systems that have invested in genomics will have access. Ledbetter agreed that it will be a challenge, but he noted that the population primarily served by Geisinger is disadvantaged by multiple criteria (e.g., predominantly of low socioeconomic status with an increased incidence of health problems such as obesity and diabetes).

Current Missed Opportunities

Ledbetter highlighted two missed opportunities that are affecting efforts to implement and integrate genomics into clinical care.

Lost Genomes

Although trio genome sequencing is now being done (and reimbursed by many payers) for diagnosis of NICU patients and pediatric neuro-developmental disorders, Ledbetter explained that "the parental genomes are just used for reference to interpret the variant of the child." There is no further interpretation of the parental genomes, which he said could be used to inform parents of their own potential health risks or for pharmaco-

---

[1] See https://guardian-study.org/ (accessed January 20, 2023).

[2] Trio exome sequencing is used to identify genetic alterations by sequencing not only the patient, but also their parents (Hebert et al., 2022).

genomics, for example. Further, he said the child's genome is only used to address the acute diagnostic question. These "lost genomes" are not retained, or are stored and forgotten, when they could be made available for interpretation and to inform care throughout the life span of the child and the parents.

The United States Lags on Implementation

Although the development of genomic technology is advancing rapidly in the United States, the country lags far behind the UK in the implementation of genomics in care, Ledbetter said. For example, the UK NHS and Genomics England launched the 100,000 Genomes Project in 2013 to study the role of genes in rare diseases and cancer. In 2022, the UK NHS and the Our Future Health program announced a 5-million-participant clinical study of the role of polygenic risk scores in preventing common adult diseases. The UK NHS established Health Education England, Ledbetter noted, which is dedicated to health care workforce training, including educating clinicians about genomics.

Genomics England and other initiatives are evidence of the political will in the UK for the implementation of genomics in health care, Wordsworth said, and certainly having a single health care system helps. However, she added, the success can also be attributed to the significant support and effort from academics, clinicians, and others who are eager to see genomics implemented. "A lot of the work that has been done has been done in people's spare time just to help the initiative move forward," she said.

Ledbetter suggested that the roundtable could convene a workshop in London, inviting leaders of the UK NHS and the leadership of NIH, CMS, and the U.S. Department of Health and Human Services (HHS). He acknowledged that the United States and UK have very different payment systems but said that HHS needs to bring NIH and CMS together to discuss what evidence CMS needs NIH to generate to support CMS coverage of whole genome sequencing for the desired range of circumstances.

GENOMICS AT PROVIDENCE: A VISION FOR THE FUTURE

As an example of how organizations are looking to realize the promise of genomics in precision care, Amy Compton-Phillips, president and chief clinical officer at Press Gainey, presented an overview of the vision for genomics at Providence, a community-based health care organization.[3]

---

[3] Compton-Phillips was president of clinical care at Providence until September 2022, joining Press Gainey in October 2022, just prior to the workshop. She spoke from her experience at Providence.

Providence believes "Genomics can be a gateway to creating whole-person care and wellness by improving prevention, early diagnosis, and treatment," she said. The goal at Providence is to accelerate the translation of evidence-based genomics from research to practice, embedding genomics innovation into patient care.

Pathways to Using Genomics in Clinical Practice

The Providence Genomics Lab was established in 2014, around the time that next-generation sequencing of tumors was beginning to be used to guide cancer treatment decisions. With philanthropic funding, Providence acquired Illumina sequencing instrumentation and has expanded over time to provide deep tumor sequencing services to all 52 Providence hospitals in multiple western U.S. states as part of its GenOmic Cancer Profiling program. A virtual tumor board was established to ensure that all clinicians were able to use the sequencing data provided to inform their treatment decisions.

Providence has been integrating genomic screening tools at the point of care where individuals would be most interested in being screened. For example, the CARE program uses online or phone-based surveys to identify women coming in for mammography who might also benefit from genetic testing for increased risk of breast cancer. Compton-Phillips said this program has been highly effective and has thus far identified about 60,000 women as high risk. Of those who were then sent for *BRCA* gene testing, about 26,000 were positive.

Providence is also expanding to provide liquid biopsy services using the Galleri multicancer early detection blood test. A study is under way to conduct 5,000 tests in the primary care setting. There are many questions to be answered before this approach can be widely implemented, Compton-Phillips said. For example, if a patient's liquid biopsy indicates they are at risk for colon cancer, but they already had a colonoscopy last year, what actions should be taken (e.g., another colonoscopy, CT scan, or wait)?

Finally, Geno4ME is Providence's whole genome sequencing program.[4] The program launched targeting higher-risk populations with a focus on underrepresented populations, Compton-Phillips said. Currently over 2,000 people have been enrolled, about 48 percent of whom identify as a person of color or member of a minority group. A challenge now is returning contextualized information to participants' primary care providers in a way that is actionable, such as embedding pharmacogenomics information into the EHR. Efforts are under way to launch EHR pharmacogenomics

---

[4]For more information on Geno4ME, see https://www.geno4me.org/en/home (accessed January 5, 2023).

decision support tools, and there is also a hotline number for providers or patients to speak with a medical geneticist.

"We really haven't harnessed the capacity of the technology yet," Compton-Phillips said. There are many hurdles to be addressed in adopting genomics into routine care, "but we're not going to learn how to do it until we start," she said.

Other Potential Considerations for the Future

Participants raised several other issues to be addressed as genomics is more broadly adopted in the coming years. Maxwell highlighted the need to ensure the necessary computing infrastructure is in place to both store the vast amounts of genomic data and to enable reanalysis. While an individual's genome sequence is static, the interpretation is dynamic, and there must be capability to reanalyze genomes, she said. Providence is building the tools to support the future of genomics, Compton-Phillips said. Whole genome sequencing at Providence is currently being conducted as implementation research. There is a new tool that facilitates electronic enrollment of participants. A "dynamic e-consent platform" allows participants to select how their data can be used and to update their consent to use their data at any time in the future. Providence has partnered with Microsoft to develop structured data cloud storage that is indexed to enable genomic information to be requeried (Microsoft does not have access to participant data). Following on the comment by Ledbetter, Compton-Phillips said that Providence does requery the patient's genome as part of their annual physical. She said Providence is hoping that providing cutting-edge genomics as part of primary care will differentiate them in the health care market.

What lessons, Feero asked, from these ongoing efforts to implement DNA sequencing in clinical care could be applied to facilitate more rapid uptake of other molecular diagnostics in the future, such as RNA sequencing, DNA methylation analysis, proteomics, metabolomics, epigenetics, and microbiome analysis? The focus needs to be not only on collecting data but on how to put these data into practice, Compton-Phillips said. Providence is taking an implementation science approach to answering key questions such as how to build trust with communities of color so they share their data, which can then be used to improve their care, she said, or how to share data about genomic variants with clinicians and patients in a meaningful, actionable way. There is still much to be elucidated about what methylation patterns and microbiome profiles mean for an individual's health, for example. But there are lessons that can be learned now such as how to manage the volumes of molecular data collected for an individual patient and put it in context for their health, Compton-Phillips said.

WORKSHOP REFLECTIONS

Martin summarized her key lessons from each of the panel sessions (Box 7-2). As discussed throughout the workshop, the use of genomic information in clinical care today is primarily reactive, and there are bottlenecks that obstruct access to genomics, Martin said. The hope for the future is for genomic information to be "readily and routinely available and accessible" for use by providers and patients, and there was much discussion about the need for improved integration of genomic data into the EHR in a manner that enables access, interrogation, and sharing. Many of the challenges that impede equitable access to precision health care are not unique from other areas of health care, she said, but the field has not adequately addressed them through education, better resources, or efforts to build trust. Martin highlighted opportunities to integrate genomics into routine clinical care across the life span in areas such as prevention, early detection, clinical diagnosis, treatment, and surveillance.

Recurrent themes across the workshop discussions, as summarized by Martin, included opportunities for

- equitable adoption of genomics at the population level;
- improved education and training of providers and the public;
- less reliance on genetics specialty clinics and greater support for integration of genetics into routine care;
- EHR-integrated clinical decision support tools; and
- engagement of all interested parties in realizing the potential of genomics in precision health care, including patients, their families, providers, payers, the public, and others.

The discussion indicated that the evolution of genetic testing to a single genetic test (a whole genome sequence) could eliminate many of the implementation challenges and barriers discussed by panelists throughout the workshop, but there is still much work to be done to realize the potential of genomic information for the practice of medicine and the delivery of precision health care, Martin said. She reiterated the point by Henley that patients are caught up in a system where valuable time is being wasted having the same discussions year after year, and restated Henley's appeal that it is time to "stop talking about changing the system" and take the actions needed to actually do it.

BOX 7-2
Workshop Reflections as Presented by Christa Martin

Improving Health Through Genomics
- The genomics dream is "a genome for everyone who wants one." (Ashley)
- Patients and families need to be at the center. (Ashley)
- There is a disconnection between the advancement of genomic diagnostics and therapeutics and recognition by payers of the value of implementing genomics for patient health. (Ashley)
- Progress toward the dream of a genome for all who want one (Ashley):
  - Cost: significant reduction over the past 2 decades—originally costing $100 million for a complete sequence and now anticipated to be approaching $100–$200 for a laboratory to sequence a complete genome.
  - Accuracy: significant improvements in the ability to quantify the genome over the past decade have been made, but greater accuracy is still needed.
  - Speed: dramatically improved since the inception of genome sequencing—from longer than 1,000 hours to the ability to provide results in less than 8 hours.
  - Implementation and integration: many challenges persist.

Enabling Patients to Benefit from Genomics
- Genomic testing is currently complex, time consuming, and costly. (Radford)
  - Explore how to streamline and make more patient centered the pathways of diagnosis and care planning. (Radford)
  - Support is needed for patients and their families across the life span. (Goto)
- Recognize the effect of racism and biases in the clinic. (Norris)
- Provide materials that are accessible in plain language. (Henley, Norris, Radford)
- Promote consistency in care by increasing clinicians' understanding of genomic conditions. Do not place the onus on the patient. (Goto)

Building an Equitable Precision Health Care System
- Recognize that medical mistrust is not a condition that needs to be cured; it is an adaptive response to historical mistreatment. (Baker)
- Dismantle racism to overcome barriers to access. (Wilkins)
- Create an equitable precision health care system:
  - Fund research to fill reference data gaps. (Wilkins)
  - Acknowledge that some racial and ethnic groups benefit less from precision medicine. (Wilkins)
  - Include social and structural determinants of health data. (Wilkins)
  - Center the needs and preferences of minoritized communities. (Wilkins)
  - Offer trainings and resources on working with diverse populations including the LGBTQ community. (Baker)
  - Build trust in health and science. (Baker, Wilkins)

continued

BOX 7-2 Continued

Logistical Challenges and Opportunities

- Follow-up on the genetics test result will soon be the rate-limiting step (rather than the test cost). (Ashley, Hilborne)
- Think about genetics as a tool to inform primary care decision making. (Massart)
- Consider different implementation models to better integrate and scale genomics in primary care settings. (Massart)
- The goal is for seamless integration of genetics into family medicine. (Massart)
- Rethink payment and reimbursement models for genomics to enable broad patient access. (Massart)
- Consider education and training opportunities. (Hilborne, Massart)
- Move from discussion to action, making real change to the system so patients' valuable time is not wasted. (Henley)

System-Level Challenges and Opportunities

- For primary care physicians to implement genomics in the clinic they need more time and a new payment and care delivery paradigm that incentivizes patient care and outcomes. (Zazove)
- Educate the public about the health benefits of genomic technologies. (Cunningham)
- Facilitate trust in science and medicine by partnering with community leaders. (Cunningham)
- Genomic data need to be "intelligible, actionable, and live." (Kaul)
- EHR-integrated clinical decision support tools are needed to enable genomics as part of routine care. (Kaul)
- Recognize that providers have various levels of expertise, and make the system fit this rather than the other way around. (Maxwell)

This list is the rapporteurs' summary of points made by the individual speakers identified, and the statements have not been endorsed or verified by the National Academies of Sciences, Engineering, and Medicine. They are not intended to reflect a consensus among workshop participants.

References

Ashley, E. A. 2016. Towards precision medicine. *Nature Reviews Genetics* 17(9):507-522.

Bagenstos, S. R. 2016. The disability cliff. *Democracy* 35:55-67.

Carlos, R. C., S. Obeng-Gyasi, S. W. Cole, B. J. Zebrack, E. D. Pisano, M. A. Troester, L. Timsina, L. I. Wagner, J. A. Steingrimsson, I. Gareen, C. I. Lee, A. S. Adams, and C. H. Wilkins. 2022. Linking structural racism and discrimination and breast cancer outcomes: A social genomics approach. *Journal of Clinical Oncology* 40(13):1407-1413.

Chan, S. L., H. Z. W. Liew, F. Nguyen, J. Thumboo, W. C. Chow, and C. Sung C. 2021. Prescription patterns of outpatients and the potential of multiplexed pharmacogenomic testing. *British Journal of Clinical Pharmacology* 87(3):886-894.

Chanfreau-Coffinier, C., L. E. Hull, J. A. Lynch, S. L. DuVall, S. M. Damrauer, F. E. Cunningham, B. F. Voight, M. E. Matheny, D. W. Oslin, M. S. Icardi, and S. Tuteja. 2019. Projected prevalence of actionable pharmacogenetic variants and level A drugs prescribed among U.S. Veterans Health Administration pharmacy users. *Journal of the American Medical Association Network Open* 2(6):e195345.

Dewey, F. E., M. E. Grove, C. Pan, B. A. Goldstein, J. A. Bernstein, H. Chaib, J. D. Merker, R. L. Goldfeder, G. M. Enns, S. P. David, N. Pakdaman, K. E. Ormond, C. Caleshu, K. Kingham, T. E. Klein, M. Whirl-Carrillo, K. Sakamoto, M. T. Wheeler, A. J. Butte, J. M. Ford, L. Boxer, J. P. Ioannidis, A. C. Yeung, R. B. Altman, T. L. Assimes, M. Snyder, E. A. Ashley, and T. Quertermous. 2014. Clinical interpretation and implications of whole-genome sequencing. *Journal of the American Medical Association* 311(10):1035-1045.

Dunnenberger, H. M., K. R. Crews, J. M. Hoffman, K. E. Caudle, U. Broeckel, S. C. Howard, R. J. Hunkler, T. E. Klein, W. E. Evans, and M. V. Relling. 2015. Preemptive clinical pharmacogenetics implementation: Current programs in five U.S. medical centers. *Annual Review of Pharmacology and Toxicology* 55:89-106.

Fleisher, L. A., and J. D. Blum. 2022. A Vision of Medicare coverage for new and emerging technologies—A consistent process to foster innovation and promote value. *Journal of the American Medical Association Internal Medicine*. Published online October 12, 2022.

Fridley, B. L., G. D. Jenkins, A. Batzler, L. Wang, Y. Ji, F. Li, and R. M. Weinshilboum. 2010. Multivariate models to detect genomic signatures for a class of drugs: Application to thiopurines pharmacogenomics. *Pharmacogenomics Journal* 12:105-110.

Gorzynski, J. E., S. D. Goenka, K. Shafin, T. D. Jensen, D. G. Fisk, M. E. Grove, E. Spiteri, T. Pesout, J. Monlong, G. Baid, J. A. Bernstein, S. Ceresnak, P. C. Chang, J. W. Christle, H. Chubb, K. P. Dalton, K. Dunn, D. R. Garalde, J. Guillory, J. W. Knowles, A. Kolesnikov, M. Ma, T. Moscarello, M. Nattestad, M. Perez, M. R. Z. Ruzhnikov, M. Samadi, A. Setia, C. Wright, C. J. Wusthoff, K. Xiong, T. Zhu, M. Jain, F. J. Sedlazeck, A. Carroll, B. Paten, and E. A. Ashley. 2022. Ultrarapid nanopore genome sequencing in a critical care setting. *New England Journal of Medicine* 386(7):700-702.

Green, E. 2023. *Exome.* genome.gov/genetics-glossary/Exome (accessed February 6, 2023).

Haidar, C. E., K. R. Crews, J. M. Hoffman, M. V. Relling, and K. E. Caudle. 2022. Advancing pharmacogenomics from single-gene to preemptive testing. *Annual Review of Genomics and Human Genetics* 23:449-473.

Halley, M. C., E. A. Ashley, and H. K. Tabor. 2022a. Supporting undiagnosed participants when clinical genomics studies end. *Nature Genetics* 54(8):1063-1065.

Halley, M. C., H. S. Smith, E. A. Ashley, A. J. Goldenberg, and H. K. Tabor. 2022b. A call for an integrated approach to improve efficiency, equity, and sustainability in rare disease research in the United States. *Nature Genetics* 54(3):219-222.

Hebert, A., A. Simons, J. H. M. Schuurs-Hoeijmakers, H. J. P. M. Koenen, E. Zonneveld-Huijssoon, S. S. V. Henriet, E. J. H. Schatorjé, E. P. A. H. Hoppenreijs, E. K. S. M. Leenders, E. J. M. Janssen, G. W. E. Santen, S. A. de Munnik, S. V. van Reijmersdal, E. van Rijssen, S. Kersten, M. G. Netea, R. L. Smeets, F. L. van de Veerdonk, A. Hoischen, and C. I. van der Made. 2022. Trio-based whole exome sequencing in patients with suspected sporadic inborn errors of immunity: A retrospective cohort study. *eLife* 11:e78469.

Hoffman, J. M., C. E. Haidar, M. R. Wilkinson, K. R. Crews, D. K. Baker, N. M. Kornegay, W. Yang, C. H. Pui, U. M. Reiss, A. H. Gaur, S. C. Howard, W. E. Evans, U. Broeckel, and M. V. Relling. 2014. PG4KDS: A model for the clinical implementation of pre-emptive pharmacogenetics. *American Journal of Medical Genetics Part C: Seminars in Medical Genetics* 166C(1):45-55.

Ibañez, K., J. Polke, R. T. Hagelstrom, E. Dolzhenko, D. Pasko, E. R. A. Thomas, L. C. Daugherty, D. Kasperaviciute, K. R. Smith; WGS for Neurological Diseases Group, Z. C. Deans, S. Hill, T. Fowler, R. H. Scott, J. Hardy, P. F. Chinnery, H. Houlden, A. Rendon, M. J. Caulfield, M. A. Eberle, R. J. Taft, A. Tucci, and the Genomics England Research Consortium. 2022. Whole genome sequencing for the diagnosis of neurological repeat expansion disorders in the UK: A retrospective diagnostic accuracy and prospective clinical validation study. *Lancet Neurology* 21(3):234-245.

IOM (Institute of Medicine). 2003. *Unequal treatment: Confronting racial and ethnic disparities in health care.* Washington, DC: The National Academies Press.

IOM. 2013. *The economics of genomic medicine: Workshop summary.* Washington, DC: The National Academies Press.

IOM and NRC (National Research Council). 2011. *Direct-to-consumer genetic testing: Summary of a workshop.* Washington, DC: The National Academies Press.

Kim, D. S., L. Wiel, and E. A. Ashley. 2022. Mind the gap: The complete human genome unlocks benefits for clinical genomics. *Clinical Chemistry*, hvac133.

Kimpton, J. E., I. M. Carey, C. J. D. Threapleton, A. Robinson, T. Harris, D. G. Cook, S. DeWilde, and E. H. Baker. 2019. Longitudinal exposure of English primary care patients to pharmacogenomic drugs: An analysis to inform design of pre-emptive pharmacogenomic testing. *British Journal of Clinical Pharmacology* 85(12):2734-2746.

Kuch, W., C. Rinner, W. Gall, and M. Samwald. 2016. How many patients could benefit from pre-emptive pharmacogenomic testing and decision support? A retrospective study based on nationwide Austrian claims data. *Studies in Health Technology and Informatics* 223:253-258.

Kwon, D. H., H. T. Borno, H. H. Cheng, A. Y. Zhou, and E. J. Small. 2020. Ethnic disparities among men with prostate cancer undergoing germline testing. *Urologic Oncology* 38(3):80.e1-80.e7.

Lewis, A. C. F., S. J. Molina, P. S. Appelbaum, B. Dauda, A. Di Rienzo, A. Fuentes, S. M. Fullerton, N. A. Garrison, N. Ghosh, E. M. Hammonds, D. S. Jones, E. E. Kenny, P. Kraft, S. S. Lee, M. Mauro, J. Novembre, A. Panofsky, M. Sohail, B. M. Neale, and D. S. Allen. 2022. Getting genetic ancestry right for science and society. *Science* 376(6590):250-252.

Miller, N. A., E. G. Farrow, M. Gibson, L. K. Willig, G. Twist, B. Yoo, T. Marrs, S. Corder, L. Krivohlavek, A. Walter, J. E. Petrikin, C. J. Saunders, I. Thiffault, S. E. Soden, L. D. Smith, D. L. Dinwiddie, S. Herd, J. A. Cakici, S. Catreux, M. Ruehle, and S. F. Kingsmore. 2015. A 26-hour system of highly sensitive whole genome sequencing for emergency management of genetic diseases. *Genome Medicine* 7:100.

Moore, G. 1965. Cramming more components onto integrated circuits. *Electronics* 38(8).

NASEM (National Academies of Sciences, Engineering, and Medicine). 2018. *Implementing and evaluating genomic screening programs in health care systems: Proceedings of a workshop*. Washington, DC: The National Academies Press.

NASEM. 2022. *Measuring sex, gender identity, and sexual orientation*. Washington, DC: The National Academies Press.

Ndugga-Kabuye, M. K., and R. B. Issaka. 2019. Inequities in multi-gene hereditary cancer testing: Lower diagnostic yield and higher VUS rate in individuals who identify as Hispanic, African, or Asian and Pacific Islander as compared to European. *Familial Cancer* 18(4):465-469.

Nguyen, J. Q., K. R. Crews, B. T. Moore, N. M. Krnegay, D. K. Baker, M. Hasan, P. K. Campbell, S. M. Dean, M. V. Relling, J. M. Hoffman, and C. E. Haidar. 2022. Clinician adherence to pharmacogenomics prescribing recommendations in clinical decision support alerts. *Journal of the American Medical Informatics Association* ocac187.

Popejoy, A. B., and S. M. Fullerton. 2016. Genomics is failing on diversity. *Nature* 538(7624):161-164.

Priest, J. R., S. R. Ceresnak, F. E. Dewey, L. E. Malloy-Walton, K. Dunn, M. E. Grove, M. V. Perez, K. Maeda, A. M. Dubin, and E. A. Ashley. 2014. Molecular diagnosis of long QT syndrome at 10 days of life by rapid whole genome sequencing. *Heart Rhythm* 11(10):1707-1713.

Quansah, E., and N. W. McGregor. 2018. Towards diversity in genomics: The emergence of neurogenomics in Africa? *Genomics* 110(1):1-9.

Roberts, M. E., L. R. Susswein, W. J. Cheng, N. J. Carter, A. C. Carter, R. T. Klein, K. S. Hruska, and M. L. Marshall. 2020. Ancestry-specific hereditary cancer panel yields: Moving toward more personalized risk assessment. *Journal of Genetic Counseling* 29(4):598-606.

Samwald, M., H. Xu, K. Blagec, P. E. Empey, D. C. Malone, S. M. Ahmed, P. Ryan, S. Hofer, and R. D. Boyce. 2016. Incidence of exposure of patients in the United States to multiple drugs for which pharmacogenomic guidelines are available. *PLoS One* 11(10):e0164972.

Saunders, C. J., N. A. Miller, S. E. Soden, D. L. Dinwiddie, A. Noll, N. A. Alnadi, N. Andraws, M. L. Patterson, L. A. Krivohlavek, J. Fellis, S. Humphray, P. Saffrey, Z. Kingsbury, J. C. Weir, J. Betley, R. J. Grocock, E. H. Margulies, E. G. Farrow, M. Artman, N. P. Safina, J. E. Petrikin, K. P. Hall, and S. F. Kingsmore. 2012. Rapid whole-genome sequencing for genetic disease diagnosis in neonatal intensive care units. *Science Translational Medicine* 4(154):154ra135.

Schildcrout, J. S., J. C. Denny, E. Bowton, W. Gregg, J.M. Pully, M. A. Basford, J. D. Cowan, H. Xu, A. H. Ramirez, D. C. Crawford, M. D. Ritchie, J. F. Peterson, D. R. Masys, R. A. Wilke, and D. M. Roden. 2012. Optimizing drug outcomes through pharmacogenetics: A case for preemptive genotyping. *Clinical Pharmacology & Therapeutics* 92(2):235-242.

Shchelochkov, O. A. 2023. *Gigabase (GB).* https://www.genome.gov/genetics-glossary/Gigabase#:~:text=A%20gigabase%20(abbreviated%20Gb)%20is,equal%20to%20 1%20billion%20bases (accessed February 3, 2023).

Sirugo, G., S. M. Williams, and S. A. Tishkoff. 2019. The missing diversity in human genetic studies. *Cell* 177(1):26-31.

Slatko, B. E., A. F. Gardner, and F. M. Ausubel. 2018. Overview of next-generation sequencing technologies. *Current Protocols in Molecular Biology* 122(1):e59.

Spencer, J. 2019. *How much is the average PTO in the U.S.?* https://www.zenefits.com/workest/how-much-is-average-pto-in-the-us/ (accessed December 29, 2022).

Splinter, K., D. R. Adams, C. A. Bacino, H. J. Bellen, J. A. Bernstein, A. M. Cheatle-Jarvela, C. M. Eng, C. Esteves, W. A. Gahl, R. Hamid, H. J. Jacob, B. Kikani, D. M. Koeller, I. S. Kohane, B. H. Lee, J. Loscalzo, X. Luo, A. T. McCray, T. O. Metz, J. J. Mulvihill, S. F. Nelson, C. G. S. Palmer, J. A. Phillips 3rd, L. Pick, J. H. Postlethwait, C. Reuter, V. Shashi, D. A. Sweetser, C. J. Tifft, N. M. Walley, M. F. Wangler, M. Westerfield, M. T. Wheeler, A. L. Wise, E. A. Worthey, S. Yamamoto, and E. A. Ashley; for the Undiagnosed Diseases Network. 2018. Effect of genetic diagnosis on patients with previously undiagnosed disease. *New England Journal of Medicine* 379(22):2131-2139.

Zeitler, E. P., L. G. Gilstrap, M. Coylewright, D. J. Slotwiner, C. H. Colla, and S. M. Al-Khatib. 2022. Coverage with evidence development: Where are we now? *American Journal of Managed Care* 28(8):382-389.

Appendix A

Workshop Agenda

Keck Building of the National Academies and by webcast
Wednesday, October 12, 2022
10:30 AM – 5:50 PM ET

SESSION I: OPENING REMARKS AND KEYNOTE PRESENTATION

Moderator: Sarah Wordsworth, Professor and University Lecturer;
               Health Economics Research Centre, Nuffield Department
               of Population Health, University of Oxford

10:30 AM ET   **Welcoming Remarks**
               Michelle Penny, *Roundtable Cochair*
               Executive Vice President, Research and Development
               Embark, Inc.

               Greg Feero, *Roundtable Cochair*
               Representing the *Journal of the American Medical
                   Association*
               Professor, Department of Community and Family
                   Medicine, Geisel School of Medicine
               Faculty, Maine Dartmouth Family Medicine Residency
                   Program

10:40–10:50 AM **Introduction and Charge to the Workshop Speakers
and Participants**
Mira Irons, *Workshop Planning Committee Cochair*
President & CEO
College of Physicians of Philadelphia

Christa Martin, *Workshop Planning Committee
Cochair*
Chief Scientific Officer, Geisinger
Professor and Director, Autism & Developmental
Medical Institute

10:50–11:15 AM **Keynote**
Euan Ashley
Associate Dean, School of Medicine
Roger and Joelle Burnell Professor of Genomics and
Precision Health
Professor of Medicine, Genetics, Biomedical Data
Science, & Pathology
Stanford University

SESSION II: WHAT DO PATIENTS NEED
AS GENOMICS MOVES INTO CLINICAL CARE?

Comoderators: Gwen Darien, Executive Vice President for Patient
Advocacy and Engagement, National Patient Advocate
Foundation and Candace Henley, Founder/Chief
Surviving Officer, The Blue Hat Foundation

Objectives   • Explore how patients assess and act upon genetic
risk information they receive from genomic
applications that may change over time (e.g.,
consumer genetic testing, polygenic risk scores,
prenatal testing).
• Examine what patients may need to make informed
decisions surrounding genetic testing and follow-up
care.

11:15–11:30 AM **Keri Norris**
Vice President of Health Equity, Diversity, and Inclusion
National Hemophilia Foundation

11:30–11:45 AM   **Greta Goto**
Founding Member
Prader-Willi Syndrome Alaska Parent Group
Cochair, Community Engagement in Genomics
     Working Group
NHGRI

11:45–12:00 PM   **Cristi Radford**
Product Director
Optum

12:00–12:25 PM   **Panel Discussion**

12:25–1:25 PM   **Break**

SESSION III: WHAT WILL IT TAKE TO BUILD AN EQUITABLE PRECISION HEALTH CARE SYSTEM?

Moderator: Gabriel Lázaro-Muñoz, Assistant Professor of Psychiatry, Member of HMS Center for Bioethics, Harvard Medical School

Objectives
- Discuss what an equitable precision health care system is and what it would take to deliver on this promise for patients and clinicians.
- Explore barriers that could be broken down to build an equitable precision health care system (e.g., access to precision health tools and clinician effectiveness in using those tools).
- Examine opportunities for improving implementation by engaging underserved and diverse communities.

1:25–1:40 PM   **Kellan Baker**
Executive Director and Chief Learning Officer
Whitman-Walker Institute

1:40–1:55 PM   **Consuelo Wilkins**
Professor of Medicine
Senior Vice President and Senior Associate Dean, for
     Health Equity and Inclusive Excellence
Engagement Core Director, All of Us Research Program
Vanderbilt University Medical Center

1:55–2:10 PM   **Mary Relling**
                   Coinvestigator and Cofounder, Clinical
                        Pharmacogenetics Implementation Consortium
                   Endowed Chair, Pharmaceutical Sciences Department
                   St. Jude Children's Research Hospital

2:10–2:35 PM   **Panel Discussion**

SESSION IV: WHAT GENETIC TESTING LOGISTICS ISSUES NEED TO BE ADDRESSED?

Moderator: Victoria Pratt, Vice President, Molecular Diagnostic
                   Quality Assessments, Optum Genomics

Objectives   • Examine and compare what evidence (e.g., clinical
                     validity and clinical utility) means in the context
                     of insurance companies, the clinical setting, and
                     laboratories creating genetic tests.
                   • Understand how patients, payers, and clinical
                     providers assess the value and benefits of genomic
                     screening and diagnostic testing.

2:35–2:50 PM ET   **Lee Hilborne**
                   Medical Director
                   Quest Diagnostics
                   Professor of Pathology and Laboratory Medicine
                   David Geffen School of Medicine
                   University of California, Los Angeles

2:50–3:05 PM   **Mylynda Massart**
                   Assistant Professor of Family Medicine
                   Department of Family Medicine
                   University of Pittsburgh
                   Founder and Director, UPMC Primary Care Precision
                        Medicine Center
                   Chair of Family Medicine, UPMC Magee Women's
                        Hospital

3:05–3:20 PM   **Bruce Quinn**
                   Principal
                   Bruce Quinn Associates LLC

3:20–3:45 PM   **Panel Discussion**

3:45–4:05 PM   Break

SESSION V: WHAT ARE THE SYSTEM-LEVEL CHALLENGES AND OPPORTUNITIES?

Moderator: W. Gregory Feero, Professor, Department of Community and Family Medicine, Geisel School of Medicine; Faculty, Maine Dartmouth Family Medicine Residency Program

Objectives
- Examine system-level barriers to widespread adoption of genomics and precision health care including data integration, cost and payment, and leadership buy-in.
- Discuss what non-geneticist clinicians may need in order to adopt genetic testing in clinical care.

4:05–4:25 PM ET Initial Remarks (5 min. each)

Philip Zazove
Professor Emeritus
Department of Family Medicine
University of Michigan

Tshaka Cunningham
Chief Scientific Officer and Cofounder
Polaris Genomics
Executive Director
Faith Based Genetic Research Institute

Karen Kaul
Chair, Department of Pathology and Laboratory Medicine
Duckworth Family Chair
NorthShore University HealthSystem
Clinical Professor of Pathology
University of Chicago Pritzker School of Medicine

Kara Maxwell
Assistant Professor of Medicine
Perelman School of Medicine
University of Pennsylvania

4:25–5:10 PM   **Panel Discussion**

SESSION VI: WHAT WILL GENOMICS ADOPTION LOOK LIKE IN THE FUTURE?

Moderator:	Mira Irons, President and CEO, College of Physicians of Philadelphia

Objective

- Explore what adoption may look like in the next 10-20 years – how clinicians will be ordering genetic testing, accessing and interpreting results, and using genetic data in routine health care.
- Explore how individuals will access their results and act on them as part of their health care.

5:10–5:35 PM   **Moderated Discussion**
Amy Compton-Phillips
President and Chief Clinical Officer
Press Ganey consulting division

David H. Ledbetter
Chief Clinical and Research Officer
Unified Patient Network, Inc.
Professor, Department of Psychiatry
University of Florida

5:35–5:50 PM   **Wrap-Up**
Mira Irons, *Workshop Planning Committee Cochair*
President and CEO
College of Physicians of Philadelphia

Christa Martin, *Workshop Planning Committee Cochair*
Chief Scientific Officer, Geisinger
Professor and Director, Autism & Developmental
   Medical Institute

5:50 PM   **Adjourn**

Appendix B

Speaker Biographies

Euan Ashley, B.Sc., M.B. Ch.B., FRCP, D.Phil., FAHA, FACC, FES, is associate dean and professor of medicine and genetics at Stanford University in California. Over the last decade his team has focused on the application of the human genome to medicine. He was recognized by the Obama White House for his contributions to personalized medicine and awarded the American Heart Association Medal of Honor for Genomic and Precision Medicine. His book, *The Genome Odyssey—Medical Mysteries and the Incredible Quest to Solve Them*, was released in 2021. He is cofounder of three companies: Personalis, DeepCell, and SVEXA.

Kellan Baker, Ph.D., M.P.H., M.A., is the Executive Director of Whitman-Walker Institute, the research, policy, and education arm of Whitman-Walker, a community health system in Washington, D.C., that also includes Whitman-Walker Health, a Federally Qualified Health Center. Kellan is a health services researcher, educator, and health policy professional with wide expertise in health equity research and policy, particularly with regard to LGBTQ populations. He is a frequent advisor for government and private entities, and he currently serves as an appointed member of a National Academy of Sciences consensus study committee that developed standards for the collection of sex, gender identity, and sexual orientation data by the National Institutes of Health. Kellan holds appointments as affiliate faculty in the Departments of Health Policy and Management at the George Washington University and the Johns Hopkins School of Public Health, and he received his Ph.D. in health policy and management from Johns Hopkins, where he was a health policy research scholar and Centennial Scholar; an M.P.H. and

M.A. from George Washington University; and a B.A. with high honors from Swarthmore College.

Amy Compton-Phillips, M.D., is an internationally respected physician, executive, innovator, and author. In October 2022, she became chief clinical officer at Press Ganey, focusing on simplifying health and care. Until September 2022, Amy was president of clinical care at Providence, responsible for clinical operations and care, including improving health, care, and value outcomes delivered by the 52 hospitals, 1,085 clinics, and 120,000 caregivers of the $25 billion health system. She was instrumental in Providence's early adoption and scaling of technology advancing the future of health care. Before joining Providence in 2015, Dr. Compton-Phillips spent 22 years at Kaiser Permanente, moving from a frontline internist to ultimately serving as chief quality officer.

Tshaka Cunningham, Ph.D., is Cofounder and Chief Scientific Officer of Polaris Genomics Inc., an emerging biotechnology company using genomics and precision medicine to improve diagnosis and treatment of mental and behavioral health conditions. Dr. Cunningham, a graduate of Princeton University, received his Ph.D. in molecular biology from Rockefeller University and completed his postdoctoral training at the Pasteur Institute in Paris, France, and at the National Institutes of Health in Bethesda, Maryland. He previously worked at the Department of Veterans Affairs overseeing a federally funded national research program in aging and neurodegenerative disease and served as a subject matter expert for the VA's Genomic Medicine Implementation Program. Motivated by the timely need for advancements in diversity and inclusion in precision medicine while at the VA, Dr. Cunningham cofounded and serves as the Executive Director of the Faith-Based Genetic Research Institute, a community-based nonprofit organization dedicated to improving people's lives through the power of genomics and precision medicine. A leading voice in advocating for diversity and representation in the field of genomics, Dr. Cunningham also serves as a board member of the Future Kings and Queens of STEM biomedical program, a STEM-focused nonprofit organization for youth from underserved communities in the DC area.

Greta L. Goto, M.B.A., is an advocate, legal guardian, representative payee, and parent to a young adult who lives with Prader-Willi Syndrome; parent to a neurotypical young adult; and wife to an accomplished seafood quality assurance manager in Alaska. In her day job, Greta is a part-time research aide with the Alaska Center for Climate Assessment and Policy. She also serves as vice chair of the board of directors for the Bristol Bay Native Corporation and as cochair of the National Human Genome Research Institute

Community Engagement in Genomics Working Group. Her professional career is grounded in nonprofit and business administration, community outreach, research and project development, strategic planning, board, and committee work. Greta is a founding member of the Prader-Willi Syndrome Alaska Parent Group and a member of Prader-Willi Syndrome Association USA. She is a graduate of Georgetown University and received her M.B.A. from the University of Alaska Anchorage.

Lee H. Hilborne, M.D., M.P.H., is a professor of pathology and laboratory medicine at UCLA and served as a member of the American Society for Clinical Pathology Board of Directors for 18 years and was president from 2007 to 2008. He chairs the ASCP Effective Test Utilization Subcommittee and is a member of the Commissions on Membership and Public Policy. Dr. Hilborne is also Senior National Medical Director at Quest Diagnostics and has held multiple positions since joining Quest Diagnostics in 2008. For 5 years Dr. Hilborne was medical director, Southern California, before assuming the role of senior medical director within Medical Affairs. Dr. Hilborne has given hundreds of invited presentations nationally and internationally and has well over 100 publications in peer-reviewed journals. For 10 years Dr. Hilborne was Director of Quality Management Services and Associate Director at UCLA Health, responsible for, among other areas, quality of care and patient safety, medical staff functions, utilization review, and medical coding. He served on several federal committees, including Medicare's Ambulatory Payment Classification Advisory Committee and the Clinical Laboratory Improvement Advisory Committee (CLIAC) and is a current member of CLIAC. He was the American Hospital Association's representative to the AMA's CPT Editorial Panel and now serves as ASCP CPT Advisor to the AMA CPT Editorial Panel and as cochair of the Proprietary Laboratory Analysis Technical Advisory Group (PLA-TAG).

Karen Kaul, M.D., Ph.D., is chair of the Department of Pathology and Laboratory Medicine at NorthShore and is a clinical professor of pathology at the University of Chicago's Pritzker School of Medicine. Dr. Kaul is board certified in Anatomic Pathology and Molecular Genetic Pathology. Following a postdoctoral fellowship at the National Cancer Institute and pathology residency training at Northwestern, Dr. Kaul established one of the earliest molecular diagnostics laboratories in the United States; she and her lab have been deeply involved in the development of laboratory tests for cancer, heritable conditions, microbial diseases, and antimicrobial susceptibility. She has been significantly involved in education, regulation, and standardization of the practice of molecular pathology, and has served on FDA, CLIAC, Medicare Evidence Development & Coverage Advisory

Committee, and other panels, and testified before the Senate HELP committee on laboratory developed testing procedures in 2016. She is a past president of the Association for Molecular Pathology and served as Editor in Chief of the *Journal of Molecular Diagnostics* until 2010. She is the recipient of the 2008 Association for Molecular Pathology Leadership Award. She was an ELAM (Executive Leadership in Academic Medicine) fellow in 2011–2012. In 2011, she was appointed a Trustee of the American Board of Pathology (ABP) where she is involved in professional examination and certification efforts, and is the past president of the ABP. She also served on the Accreditation Council for Graduate Medical Education Residency Review Committee for Pathology and Milestones committees and currently leads the Association for Pathology Chairs GME committee. Dr. Kaul served as residency program director for 18 years and served on Residency Program Directors Section council before becoming departmental chair in 2012. As chair, she has led departmental efforts to improve laboratory efficiency and utilization and maximize the impact of the laboratory on clinical care. She continues to practice and advocate for molecular pathology.

David H. Ledbetter, Ph.D., FACMG, is Chief Clinical and Research Officer, Unified Patient Network, Inc. After serving as Executive Vice President and Founding Chief Scientific Officer at Geisinger for 10 years (2010-2021), Dr. Ledbetter assumed the role of Chief Clinical and Research Officer at Unified Patient Network, Inc., a start-up company building a massive precision medicine database across multiple health care systems linking patient EHR and other clinical data sets to clinical whole genome sequence data. Previously he held academic and leadership positions at Emory University, the University of Chicago, and Baylor College of Medicine. He is a graduate of Tulane University and earned his Ph.D. at the University of Texas-Austin. Dr. Ledbetter is an internationally recognized expert in genomics and precision medicine, with a special interest in autism and other pediatric brain disorders. After his discovery of the genetic causes of Prader-Willi syndrome (deletion chromosome 15; 1981) and Miller-Dieker syndrome (deletion or point mutation of a gene on chromosome 17; 1983) early in his career, he has focused his research efforts on discovering the genetic causes of childhood neurodevelopmental disorders such as autism, and the translation of new genomics technologies into clinically useful genetic tests for early diagnosis and intervention. At Geisinger, he led the development of the largest DNA-sequenced patient cohort in the United States, second only to the UK Biobank in the world. His current research interest includes implementation science efforts to move genomics and precision medicine into routine patient care to optimize prevention, early diagnosis, treatments, and outcomes across all clinical disease areas.

Mylynda B. Massart, M.D., Ph.D., is a board-certified family medicine physician at UPMC, and assistant professor at the University of Pittsburgh. She serves as the founder and Medical Director of the UPMC Primary Care Precision Medicine clinic, and as the Associate Director of Clinical Services for the Institute for Precision Medicine. Dr. Massart is codirector for the HUB Core over Research Inclusivity and Community Partners Core at the Clinical and Translational Science Institute (CSTI). Her research interests are in developing education in genetics and precision medicine for primary care providers and trainees and to be a research catalyst facilitating the inclusion of underrepresented populations in biomedical research. She teaches residents and medical students in her clinic and at the hospital and serves as medical director for Bethany Hospice. Currently, Dr. Massart is one of the co-investigators for the All of US Pennsylvania research project working on community education and engagement. In addition, she is working as co-investigator to create the local Discovery Biobank at the University of Pittsburgh and developing systems to return precision medicine results to providers and patients. Dr. Massart is the principal investigator for the NIH Community Engagement Alliance (CEAL) Consultative Resource (CEACR) team.

Kara Maxwell, M.D., Ph.D., is an assistant professor in the Department of Medicine, Division of Hematology/Oncology and the Department of Genetics at the University of Pennsylvania School of Medicine and a Staff Physician at the Corporal Michael Crescenz Veterans Affairs Medical Center. She completed her bachelor of science with a dual major in genetics and biochemistry at the University of Wisconsin-Madison and completed her M.D.-Ph.D. at the Weill Cornell Medical College and Rockefeller University. Dr. Maxwell performed her doctoral training with Dr. Jan Breslow at the Rockefeller University in the field of cholesterol metabolism where she cloned and characterized the mouse and human forms of *Pcsk9*. She then performed her internal medicine residency at New York Presbyterian Hospital Columbia and her hematology/oncology fellowship at the University of Pennsylvania. She subsequently completed a cancer genetics fellowship and postdoctoral training in the field of human cancer genetics at the University of Pennsylvania. Dr. Maxwell performed her postdoctoral training in the laboratory of Dr. Katherine Nathanson at Penn Medicine, focusing on cancer genetics and genomics in *BRCA*-deficient breast and ovarian cancer. Dr. Maxwell's clinical practice is in the area of cancer risk evaluation and includes medical management of a variety of cancer risk syndromes. At Penn Medicine, she is a regional referral expert for patients with Li Fraumeni Syndrome, a rare cancer risk syndrome caused by *TP53* mutations. Dr. Maxwell also codirects the Cancer Genetics Program at the Corporal Michael Crescenz Veterans Affairs Medical Center in Philadelphia where she works to provide alternative genetic testing care models to a racially diverse population of veterans. In her Veterans Affairs role, Dr. Maxwell is also an expert consultant for the National Precision Oncology Program (NPOP) where she provides consultation for implementing cancer risk and tumor genomic testing. Dr. Maxwell's laboratory studies mechanisms of tumor formation in breast and prostate cancer due to germline mutations in *TP53* and other DNA repair genes. Dr. Maxwell is a recipient of the Burroughs Wellcome Career Award for Medical Scientists and a National Cancer Institute K08 Award. She is also funded through the Prostate Cancer Foundation, the Li Fraumeni Syndrome Association, and the Basser Center for *BRCA* at Penn Medicine.

Keri Norris, Ph.D., M.P.H., MCHES, is a public health professional with extensive training and expertise in health equity, health promotion, and disease prevention at the local, state, and federal level. She has worked for some premiere public health and higher education institutions (including the Centers for Disease Control and Prevention, the Fulton DeKalb Hospital Authority, Spelman College, Agnes Scott College, Baylor University, and Morehouse School of Medicine). She is currently the Vice President of Health Equity, Diversity, and Inclusion for the National Hemophilia Foundation. She has a TEDx Talk on Hiding in Plain Sight: Health Equity and What's Missing. She is a graduate of Agnes Scott College, Morehouse School of Medicine, the University of South Carolina, and Emory University Law School. Keri serves on the board of Henry County Board of Health, Good Samaritan Health Center Atlanta, Haven of Light, International, and the advisory board of the National Coalition Against Domestic Violence. She is a member of Junior League DeKalb and Alpha Kappa Alpha Sorority, Inc.

Cristi Radford, M.S., CGC, Product Director, is responsible for overseeing the development and launch of genetic test management capabilities within Optum's laboratory benefit management solution. Previously, Radford served as Director of Genetics, Clinical Initiatives, for UnitedHealthcare, where she was responsible for developing and implementing strategies to improve access to genetic testing and services while driving affordability and member outcomes. Of note, she spearheaded the launch of Fit-at-50, a program increasing the use of direct-to-member, in-home, colorectal cancer screening for average risk members, setting a framework for precision population health programs. She also led the implementation of a rapid genetic testing program in the NICU setting, which increased the use of rapid genetic testing in NICU settings using a novel reimbursement method. Prior to joining UnitedHealth Group, Radford was Channel Development Manager at Genome Medical. Earlier in her career, Radford developed several community-based cancer risk assessment programs before transitioning into commercial molecular diagnostics in 2012 at Ambry Genetics and subsequently Invitae. Her academic roles have included positions at Vanderbilt University and Moffit Cancer Center, where she helped create and expand ICARE, as well as Johns Hopkins University. ICARE is an effort to improve access to cancer genetics expertise for patients and health care providers and includes a cancer registry. Radford holds a bachelor of science degree from the University of Georgia and a master of science degree in genetic counseling from the University of South Carolina.

Bruce Quinn, M.D., Ph.D., is an expert in Medicare policy for innovative technology. His initial career was as a full-time medical school faculty member. Armed with an M.B.A. in 2001, he shifted to a career in strategy consulting. He served as a regional Medicare Part B medical director, 2004–2008. He has worked for a global consulting firm, Accenture, as well as for two D.C.-based health policy firms. Since 2016, he has been an independent consultant primarily focused on genomics and digital technologies. His services include product planning and reimbursement pathways for innovators, as well as due diligence investigations for investors. His website on health policy and new technology, "Discoveries in Health Policy," has had over a million views, holds 2,000 articles, and has hundreds of subscribers from industry, academia, and government. Dr. Quinn is based in Los Angeles.

Mary Relling, Pharm.D., earned her undergraduate B.S. degree from the University of Arizona College of Pharmacy and her doctoral degree from the University of Utah College of Pharmacy. She completed postdoctoral fellowships with Dr. William Evans at St. Jude and with Dr. Urs Meyer at University of Basel. She joined St. Jude as a faculty member in 1988 and was chair of the Department of Pharmaceutical Sciences from 2003 to 2020. She is also a professor at the University of Tennessee in the Colleges of Medicine and Pharmacy. Her primary interests are in treatment and pharmacogenetics of childhood leukemia and clinical implementation of pharmacogenetic testing. Dr. Relling is part of NIH's Pharmacogenomics Research Network and cofounder of CPIC, the Clinical Pharmacogenetics Implementation Consortium. She has published more than 400 original scientific manuscripts. She was elected to the National Academy of Medicine (formerly Institute of Medicine) in 2009.

Consuelo H. Wilkins, M.D., MCSI, is a nationally recognized physician-scientist leader in health equity research focused on integrating social, cultural, and environmental factors into clinical and translational research. Dr. Wilkins is Senior Vice President and Senior Associate Dean for Health

Equity and Inclusive Excellence and a professor of medicine at Vanderbilt University Medical Center. Dr. Wilkins is a Principal Investigator (PI) of three NIH-funded research centers and is responsible for a portfolio of programs in response to the institutions' strategic direction for inclusion and diversity. She has also been PI of a Robert Wood Johnson Foundation Award on measuring and engendering trust in health care among African American men and a Patient-Centered Outcomes Research Award on Improving Patient Engagement and Understanding Its Impact on Research. Among Dr. Wilkins's many contributions to science is her prescient focus on engaging racial and ethnic minority communities using implementation science methodologies in the design and conduct of clinical research. She has pioneered efforts to move the academic and clinical research enterprise to transform approaches to clinical research design by embedding participant and community engagement in every aspect of biomedical discovery. An elected member of the National Academy of Medicine, she has published more than 100 papers on her research. Dr. Wilkins earned a bachelor of science in microbiology and a doctorate in medicine from Howard University and a master of science in clinical investigation from Washington University in St. Louis. She completed residency in internal medicine at Duke University Medical Center and a fellowship in geriatrics at Barnes-Jewish Hospital/Washington University Medical Center.

Philip Zazove, M.D., is professor emeritus at Michigan Medicine, University of Michigan. Dr. Zazove has profound hearing loss and is one of the first people with this to have become a physician. Dr. Zazove has been one of the pioneers researching health services and primary care for people with hearing loss—ever since he started at the University of Michigan 30 years ago. The research he has conducted, the papers he has published, the consulting he has done, and the presentations he has made at various national/international meetings have focused on health care for deaf/hard of hearing persons. Dr. Zazove has successfully managed large population-based studies with these individuals in the past. In addition, he has had an interest in primary care genomics, publishing work and completing a sabbatical in this area at University College London. Dr. Zazove graduated from Northwestern University and received his M.D. from Washington University. He completed his residency training in family medicine at the University of Utah Hospitals and a master's in business at Northwestern's Kellogg School of Business.